Food and Drug Administration's Role in Dermatology

Editor

MARKHAM C. LUKE

DERMATOLOGIC CLINICS

www.derm.theclinics.com

Consulting Editor
BRUCE H. THIERS

July 2022 • Volume 40 • Number 3

ELSEVIER

1600 John F. Kennedy Boulevard • Suite 1800 • Philadelphia, Pennsylvania, 19103-2899

http://www.theclinics.com

DERMATOLOGIC CLINICS Volume 40, Number 3
July 2022 ISSN 0733-8635, ISBN-13: 978-0-323-84969-2

Editor: Stacy Eastman
Developmental Editor: Karen Justine Solomon

Dermatologic Clinics (ISSN 0733-8635) is published quarterly by Elsevier Inc., 360 Park Avenue South, New York, NY 10010-1710. Months of publication are January, April, July, and October. Business and editorial offices: 1600 John F. Kennedy Blvd., Suite 1800, Philadelphia, PA 19103-2899. Customer service office: 11830 Westline Drive, St. Louis, MO 63146. Periodicals postage paid at New York, NY, and additional mailing offices. Subscription prices are USD 429.00 per year for US individuals, USD 1,035.00 per year for US institutions, USD 469.00 per year for Canadian individuals, USD 1,071.00 per year for Canadian institutions, USD 525.00 per year for international individuals, USD 1,071.00 per year for international institutions, USD 100.00 per year for US students/residents, USD 100.00 per year for Canadian students/residents, and USD 240 per year for international students/residents. International air speed delivery is included in all *Clinics* subscription prices. All prices are subject to change without notice. **POSTMASTER:** Send address changes to *Dermatologic Clinics*, Elsevier Health Sciences Division, Subscription Customer Service, 3251 Riverport Lane, Maryland Heights, MO 63043. **Customer Service: 1-800-654-2452 (U.S. and Canada); 314-447-8871 (outside U.S. and Canada). Fax: 314-447-8029. E-mail: journalscustomerservice-usa@elsevier.com (for print support); journalsonlinesupport-t-usa@elsevier.com (for online support).**

Reprints. For copies of 100 or more, of articles in this publication, please contact the Commercial Reprints Department, Elsevier Inc., 360 Park Avenue South, New York, New York 10010-1710. Tel.: 212-633-3874; Fax: 212-633-3820; Email: reprints@elsevier.com.

The *Dermatologic Clinics* is covered in *MEDLINE/PubMed (Index Medicus)*, *Current Contents/Clinical Medicine*, *Excerpta Medica, Chemical Abstracts,* and *ISI/BIOMED.*

Contributors

CONSULTING EDITOR

BRUCE H. THIERS, MD
Professor and Chairman Emeritus, Department of Dermatology and Dermatologic Surgery, Medical University of South Carolina, Charleston, South Carolina

EDITOR

MARKHAM C. LUKE, MD, PhD, FAAD
Director, Division of Therapeutic Performance 1, Office of Research and Standards, Office of Generic Drugs, Center for Drug Evaluation and Research, US Food and Drug Administration, Silver Spring, Maryland

AUTHORS

ROBYN BENT, RN, MS
Director, Patient Focused Drug Development, Office of Center Director, Center for Drug Evaluation and Research, US Food and Drug Administration, Silver Spring, Maryland

BRUCE A. BROD, MD, MHCI, FAAD
Chair, AADA Council on Government Affairs and Health Policy, Clinical Professor of Dermatology Perelman School of Medicine, University of Pennsylvania, Philadelphia, Pennsylvania

VANESSA L. BURROWS, PhD
History Office, US Food and Drug Administration, Silver Spring, Maryland

SELENA R. DANIELS, PharmD, PhD
Team Leader, Division of Clinical Outcome Assessment, Office of Drug Evaluation Science, Center for Drug Evaluation and Research, US Food and Drug Administration, Silver Spring, Maryland

ROSELYN E. EPPS, MD
U.S. Food and Drug Administration, Center for Drug Evaluation and Research, Division of Dermatology and Dentistry, Silver Spring, Maryland

THOMAS J. FRANZ, MD
Happy Valley, Oregon

PRIYANKA GHOSH, PhD
Senior Staff Fellow, Division of Therapeutic Performance I, Office of Research and Standards, Office of Generic Drugs, Center for Drug Evaluation and Research, US Food and Drug Administration, Silver Spring, Maryland

SHLOMIT HALACHMI, MD, PhD
Medical Officer, Center for Devices and Radiological Health, US Food and Drug Administration, Silver Spring, Maryland

LINDA M. KATZ, MD, MPH
Office of Cosmetics and Colors, Center for Food Safety and Nutrition, US Food and Drug Administration, College Park, Maryland

CINDY KORTEPETER, PharmD
Division of Pharmacovigilance, Food and Drug Administration, Center for Drug Evaluation and

Research, Office of Surveillance and Epidemiology, Silver Spring, Maryland

PAUL A. LEHMAN, MS
QPS Holdings, LLC, Newark, Delaware

FELISA S. LEWIS, MD, MPH, FAAD
Medical Reviewer, Division of Dermatology and Dentistry, Office of Inflammation and Immunology, Office of New Drugs, Center for Drug Evaluation and Research, US Food and Drug Administration, Silver Spring, Maryland

KATHLEEN M. LEWIS, JD
Office of Cosmetics and Colors, Center for Food Safety and Nutrition, US Food and Drug Administration, College Park, Maryland

MARKHAM C. LUKE, MD, PhD, FAAD
Director, Division of Therapeutic Performance 1, Office of Research and Standards, Office of Generic Drugs, Center for Drug Evaluation and Research, US Food and Drug Administration, Silver Spring, Maryland

KENDALL A. MARCUS, MD
Director, Division of Dermatology and Dentistry, Office of Inflammation and Immunology, Office of New Drugs, Center for Drug Evaluation and Research, US Food and Drug Administration, Silver Spring, Maryland

LAURA MARQUART, MD
Medical Officer, Center for Devices and Radiological Health, US Food and Drug Administration, Silver Spring, Maryland

MONICA MUÑOZ, PharmD, PhD, BCPS
Division of Pharmacovigilance, US Food and Drug Administration, Center for Drug Evaluation and Research, Office of

Surveillance and Epidemiology, Silver Spring, Maryland

ELEKTRA PAPADOPOULOS, MD, MPH
Deputy Director, Division of Clinical Outcome Assessment, Office of Drug Evaluation Science, Center for Drug Evaluation and Research, US Food and Drug Administration, Silver Spring, Maryland

TANNAZ RAMEZANLI, Pharm D, PhD
Office of Research and Standards, Office of Generic Drugs, Center for Drug Evaluation and Research, US Food and Drug Administration, Silver Spring, Maryland

SAM G. RANEY, PhD
Associate Director for Science, Office of Research and Standards, Office of Generic Drugs, Center for Drug Evaluation and Research, US Food and Drug Administration, Silver Spring, Maryland

MELISSA REYES, MD, MPH, FAAD
Division of Pharmacovigilance, Food and Drug Administration, Center for Drug Evaluation and Research, Office of Surveillance and Epidemiology, Silver Spring, Maryland; Department of Dermatology, Uniformed Services University of the Health Sciences

NAKISSA SADRIEH, PhD
Office of Cosmetics and Colors, Center for Food Safety and Nutrition, US Food and Drug Administration, College Park, Maryland

SUSAN SPENCE, PhD
Office of Cosmetics and Colors, Center for Food Safety and Nutrition, US Food and Drug Administration, College Park, Maryland

Contents

Foreword: Food and Drug Administration's Role in Dermatology   ix

Bruce A. Brod

Preface: The US Food and Drug Administration's Intersection with Dermatology   xi

Markham C. Luke

The History of Dermatology and Dermatologists at the US Food and Drug Administration   237

Vanessa L. Burrows and Markham C. Luke

In the United States, the Food and Drug Administration's (FDA's) regulatory author-ities have significantly influenced the products available to treat dermatologic conditions, but at the same time, advances in dermatology have also influenced the FDA's approach, including the agency's evaluation of risks and its' communica-tions to consumers, patients, and providers. This essay reviews significant milestones in the history of FDA's regulation of dermatologic products, with attention paid to significant products, impactful legal changes, and key personnel and organizational changes.

The Food and Drug Administration's Role in Dermatologic Drug Development   249

Felisa S. Lewis and Kendall A. Marcus

The mission of the Food and Drug Administration (FDA) is to ensure the safety and effectiveness of dermatologic drugs, as authorized by the Federal Food, Drug, and Cosmetic Act (FD&CA). In this article, we discuss how the FDA's policies and prac-tices have continued to evolve to incorporate scientific advances and to facilitate approval for dermatologic drugs in a timely manner for a broad spectrum of patients. We provide several examples to highlight areas where the Division of Dermatology and Dentistry found common ground with stakeholders to increase the therapeutic options for dermatologic patients, while still maintaining regulatory standards required for approval.

Postmarket Assessment for Drugs and Biologics Used in Dermatology and Cutaneous Adverse Drug Reactions   265

Melissa Reyes, Cindy Kortepeter, and Monica Muñoz

Postmarket surveillance is critical for the identification of rare safety risks, which are unlikely to be identified during clinical trials and the drug development program. Rare adverse drug reactions with the potential for serious outcomes, including fatal-ities, include the severe cutaneous adverse reactions of Stevens–Johnson syn-drome, toxic epidermal necrolysis, and drug reaction with eosinophilia and systemic symptoms. Dermatologists play an important role in the diagnosis of these serious drug reactions and contribute to drug safety by reporting cases of suspected cutaneous adverse drug reactions.

How Does the Food and Drug Administration Approve Topical Generic Drugs Applied to the Skin?   279

Priyanka Ghosh, Sam G. Raney, and Markham C. Luke

Approved generic drugs are therapeutically equivalent to a preidentified brand name product and are expected to have the same clinical effect and safety profile when administered to patients under conditions specified in the labeling. Availability of generic topical dermatologic drugs is expected to enhance patient access to such widely used drug products. Assessment of equivalence for a prospective generic product involves a systematic and rigorous comparative evaluation to ensure there is no significant difference in the rate and extent to which the active ingredient(s) become available at the site of action for the prospective generic and corresponding brand name product.

Dermatology Drugs for Children—U.S. Food and Drug Administration Perspective   289

Roselyn E. Epps

United States regulations benefiting pediatric drug development were not addressed until later in the twentieth century. Because of legislation, clinical trials and data analysis targeting the pediatric population have resulted in improved drug product labeling. The Best Pharmaceuticals for Children Act (BPCA), Pediatric Research Equity Act (PREA), exclusivity incentives, and newer analytical methods have increased available information regarding drug products with pediatric dermatology indications. Although legislation, clinical and pharmacological research, and analytical methods have evolved, opportunities for improvement remain. Interactive and targeted strategies are needed to allow timely drug labeling for pediatric dermatology populations.

Regulation of Medical Devices for Dermatology   297

Shlomit Halachmi and Laura Marquart

Medical devices became subject to premarket review by the Food and Drug Administration (FDA) in 1976. Devices are distinguished from drugs by the means in which they achieve their primary intended purposes. Dermatologic devices regulated by FDA range include wound care products, injectable implants, energy-based devices, and diagnostic devices. All medical devices, regardless of risk, share certain regulatory requirements to assure safety and effectiveness. Class II and Class III devices must additionally be cleared or approved by FDA before being introduced into interstate commerce.

Regulation of Cosmetics in the United States   307

Linda M. Katz, Kathleen M. Lewis, Susan Spence, and Nakissa Sadrieh

In the United States, cosmetics are regulated under the Food, Drug, and Cosmetic Act and the Fair Packaging and Labeling Act. Accordingly, cosmetic ingredients, with the exception of color additives, are not subject to premarket approval. However, they must not be adulterated or misbranded. This article describes the statutes and regulations relevant to cosmetic regulation by the Food and Drug Administration (FDA). It also describes relevant domestic programs of the FDA (Voluntary Cosmetic Registration Program, Good Manufacturing Practice guidance, Adverse Event Reporting System, Recalls) and international efforts regarding cosmetics regulation.

Cutaneous Pharmacokinetic Approaches to Compare Bioavailability and/or Bioequivalence for Topical Drug Products   319

Sam G. Raney, Priyanka Ghosh, Tannaz Ramezanli, Paul A. Lehman, and Thomas J. Franz

The evaluation of bioequivalence (BE) involves comparing the test product to its reference product in a study whose fundamental scientific principles allow one to infer the therapeutic equivalence of the products. Several test methods have been discussed by which to evaluate topical bioavailability (BA) and BE. Pharmacokinetics-based approaches characterize the rate and extent to which an active ingredient becomes available at or near its site(s) of action in the skin. Such methodologies are considered to be among the most accurate, sensitive, and reproducible approaches for determining the BA or BE of a product.

Measuring What Matters to Patients in Dermatology Drug Development: A Regulatory Perspective   333

Selena R. Daniels, Kendall A. Marcus, Robyn Bent, and Elektra Papadopoulos

Incorporating the patient voice into drug development and regulatory review process allows for the science of drug development to be more patient-centered. Dermatology is one therapeutic area where patients have the potential to provide valuable perspectives on symptoms, functional impacts, and aesthetic outcomes. Patient-reported and observer-reported outcomes play an important role in capturing concerns related to the disease or condition and its treatment. Patient experience data from well-designed trials are critical for regulatory decision-making and ultimately enable prescribers and patients to make better informed treatment decisions at the point of care.

DERMATOLOGIC CLINICS

FORTHCOMING ISSUES

October 2022
Vascular Anomalies
Lara Wine Lee and Marcelo Hochman, *Editors*

January 2023
Cutaneous Oncology Update
Stan N. Tolkachjov, *Editor*

April 2023
Diversity, Equity, and Inclusion in Dermatology
Susan C. Taylor, *Editor*

RECENT ISSUES

April 2022
Pediatric Dermatology Part II
Kelly M. Cordoro, *Editor*

January 2022
Pediatric Dermatology Part I
Kelly M. Cordoro, *Editor*

October 2021
COVID-19 and the Dermatologist
Esther E. Freeman and Devon E. McMahon, *Editors*

SERIES OF RELATED INTEREST

Medical Clinics
https://www.medical.theclinics.com/

THE CLINICS ARE AVAILABLE ONLINE!
Access your subscription at:
www.theclinics.com

Foreword

Food and Drug Administration's Role in Dermatology

Abbreviations	
AADA	American Academy of Dermatology Association
FDA	U.S. Food and Drug Administration

Prevention and treatment of skin disease are well served by the American Academy of Dermatology Association's (AADA) strong partnership with the Food and Drug Administration (FDA). For that reason, I applaud the combined leadership of Markham Luke, MD, PhD from the FDA and AADA Immediate Past President, Bruce Thiers, MD on shaping this issue of *Dermatology Clinics*, which focuses on the FDA's relationship with dermatology. The AADA and the FDA share a wide spectrum of goals when it comes to improving patient care and ensuring public safety in an ever-evolving health care system.

This important collaboration between a specialty society and a government agency can continue to streamline safe, expeditious approval of breakthrough prescription medications to treat persistent common conditions, such as vitiligo and alopecia, while using the voice of the patient in identifying gaps and challenges in care for these and other diseases as we have seen in the Patient-Focused Drug Development Initiative. With dermatology's unique insight in topical therapy, there are also opportunities to collaborate on instituting new technologies in topical therapy to meet the needs of the twenty-first century. As technology developments such as augmented intelligence often outpace our capacity to define best practices, it is essential that the AADA and FDA work together to set guardrails on appropriate use.

I hope this issue will not only prove interesting for the readers but also raise awareness of the important relationship the AADA has with the FDA. The scope of how the two groups interface is too large to cover in this publication; however, it is a noteworthy start on the path to further publications.

Bruce A. Brod, MD, MHCI, FAAD
Perelman School of Medicine, Dermatology
University of Pennsylvania
3400 Civic Center Boulevard
Building 421
Philadelphia, PA 19104

E-mail address:
bruce.brod@pennmedicine.upenn.edu

Dermatol Clin 40 (2022) ix
https://doi.org/10.1016/j.det.2022.03.004
0733-8635/22/© 2022 Published by Elsevier Inc.

Preface
The US Food and Drug Administration's Intersection with Dermatology

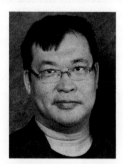

Markham C. Luke, MD, PhD, FAAD
Editor

I am writing this opinion piece and one of the forewords to this issue from the confines of my alternate workplace (my home) in the midst of the COVID-19 pandemic. My Food and Drug Administration (FDA) work allows me to do much of it from home currently due to twenty-first-century technology (ie, the Internet, thumb-sized desk-top video cameras, and collaborative work software). My coworkers and my Division have maintained a high level of work throughout and have met our work deadlines despite the pandemic. It is my assessment that this would not have been possible at the start of my career at FDA in 1998. I recall that some medical officers were still dictating their reviews to be transcribed by typists, and it was novel to have an electronic submission for a drug application. I had come to FDA from the National Institutes of Health, where I was previously serving as a Clinical Associate at the National Cancer Institute, seeing patients and conducting research in the laboratory of Dr Kim Yancey. It was a big paradigm shift for me to start as a Medical Officer reviewer for the FDA back then. I had the privilege and fortune of being hired by and working under Dr Jonathan Wilkin, an academician and dermatologist with broad interests, who took to his job as an FDA regulator with utmost enthusiasm. I recall that he was full of ideas and always thought himself fortunate to be able to work at FDA.

The FDA has grown over the years that I have worked here. It currently encompasses Center programs in foods and cosmetics (Center for Food Safety and Nutrition or CFSAN), drugs (Center for Drug Evaluation and Research or CDER), medical devices (Center for Devices and Radiologic Health or CDRH), biologics (Center for Biologics Evaluation and Research or CBER), veterinary medicine (Center for Veterinary Medicine or CVM), and tobacco (Center for Tobacco Products or CTP). In addition, there are additional centers responsible for field offices and inspections and the National Center for Toxicological Research or NCTR. Together, these entities intersect with the field of dermatology and other medical fields in multiple ways.

I am a dermatologist, board-certified, with a history of advocacy in this field as a resident and as academic faculty. Dermatology is an ideal medical field to discuss interaction with FDA. Dermatologists prescribe and use a myriad of products in the care of our patients. Skin care occurs both with and without health care worker "knowledgeable intermediaries." Various consumer and personal care products are used by the lay public to care for their skin, hair, and nails, some of which are regulated by FDA. We (my fellow article authors and I) have endeavored in this *Dermatology Clinics* issue to address broadly the various products for human use that are regulated by FDA. We attempt to anticipate some of the questions or knowledge needs about FDA that a practicing dermatologist or skin health care practitioner might have in the articles that constitute this issue.

Dermatol Clin 40 (2022) xi–xii
https://doi.org/10.1016/j.det.2022.03.003
0733-8635/22/© 2022 Published by Elsevier Inc.

We hope that you enjoy reading through the various pieces that we have assembled in this issue. For the dermatologist who is starting on her or his career, we encourage them to explore how they might contribute to the global dermatology society by considering working at FDA, perhaps as a reviewer or serving as an advisor and consultant for one of its relevant Advisory Committees should they have the qualifications and lack any conflict of interest. One of the fulfilling parts of working at FDA in my estimation is the ability to be a less conflicted observer/reviewer/gatekeeper and to work at providing consistent expert knowledge with less bias (we all have personal biases) and level-playing-field advice and decision making. This aspect, I believe, characterizes what sets apart an FDA review.

Markham C. Luke, MD, PhD, FAAD
Division of Therapeutic Performance 1
Office of Research and Standards
Office of Generic Drugs
Center for Drug Evaluation and Research
U.S. Food and Drug Administration
10903 New Hampshire Avenue
Silver Spring, MD 20993, USA

E-mail address:
markham.luke@fda.hhs.gov

The History of Dermatology and Dermatologists at the US Food and Drug Administration

Vanessa L. Burrows, PhD[a],*, Markham C. Luke, MD, PhD[b]

KEYWORDS

• Dermatology • History • Food and Drug Administration • Dermatologists • Regulation

KEY POINTS

- Dermatologic health concerns have helped contribute to transformations in US cosmetic and drug law.
- Dermatologists, together with other scientists, within and external to the agency are instrumental in the FDA's regulatory decision making.
- Dermatologic products have advanced FDA's approach to evaluating and mitigating health risks for other non-dermatologic products.

Abbreviations	
FDA	U.S. Food and Drug Administration
CDER	Center for Drug Evaluation and Research
CBER	Center for Biologics Evaluation and Research
CDRH	Center for Devices and Radiological Health
CVM	Center for Veterinary Medicine
CFSAN	Center for Food Safety and Nutrition
FFDCA	Federal Food, Drug, and Cosmetics Act

INTRODUCTION

Dermatologic therapeutics are shaped by the regulatory environment that evaluates their safety, efficacy, risks, and indications. The history of the regulation of dermatologic products is deeply embedded in the history of the US Food and Drug Administration (FDA). As FDA's regulatory authorities have evolved over time, the agency has gained new powers to advance the safety and efficacy of dermatologic products. At the same time, the FDA has adapted to innovations in the field, and changes in the marketplace and legislation, which have directly impacted the agency's legal powers. Just as the tools used by dermatologists are broad, encompassing drugs, biologics, devices, and cosmetics, the entities

This article reflects the views of the authors and should not be construed to represent FDA's views or policies. The authors do not have any applicable disclosures related to financial conflict of interest for any of the products mentioned in this article.

[a] History Office, U.S Food and Drug Administration, 10903 New Hampshire Avenue, Silver Spring, MD 20993, USA; [b] Division of Therapeutic Performance, Office of Generic Drugs, Center for Drug Evaluation and Research, U.S. Food and Drug Administration, Silver Spring, MD 20993, USA

* Corresponding author.

E-mail address: vanessa.burrows@fda.hhs.gov

Dermatol Clin 40 (2022) 237–248
https://doi.org/10.1016/j.det.2022.03.001
0733-8635/22/Published by Elsevier Inc.

that regulate these products are also broad, crossing the established Centers at the FDA and are reviewed by dermatologists and others who have come to work at FDA in various capacities and in different parts of the Agency.

FDA's regulatory authorities are given by laws passed by Congress. These laws have evolved over time to extend certain enforcement powers and scientific priorities to the agency and to define the scope of its portfolio of activities. As a result, FDA does not in itself manufacture products or, for the most part, conduct clinical research. Rather FDA reviews, inspects, provides guidance, and sets regulations for manufacturers and researchers to follow. For the purposes of this article, please reference **Table 1** whereby we list selected significant legislation that has impacted the regulation of dermatologic products at FDA.

Today, the FDA is responsible for the oversight of more than $2.8 trillion in the consumption of food, medical products, and tobacco. FDA-regulated products account for about 20 cents of every dollar spent by US consumers.[1] Just as the market of dermatologic products has grown in quantity and in complexity over time, so too have the entities at FDA that regulate these products. Since the early 1980s, FDA has been organized by Centers. Historically, most medical dermatology products have been regulated by the Center for Drug Evaluation and Research (CDER) and the Center for Devices and Radiological Health (CDRH), and their predecessors. In 2003, the review of botulinum toxin and

Table 1
Major legislative milestones that impacted the regulation of dermatology therapy

Law	Year	Regulatory Impact
Biologics Control Act	1902	Required federal licensure of biologics manufacturers and products
Federal Food and Drugs Act (aka, Pure Food and Drugs Act)	1906	Banned marketing of adulterated or misbranded food or drugs; required adherence to drug standards
Federal Food, Drug, and Cosmetic Act	1938	Mandated evidence of safety before marketing drugs; brought cosmetics and medical devices under FDA's authority; created the color certification program
Durham-Humphrey Amendments	1951	Required prescription from medical professional for certain dangerous or habit-forming drugs
1962 Drug Amendments (aka, Kefauver-Harris Amendments)	1962	In addition to safety, required drugs provide substantial evidence of efficacy from sound clinical studies before marketing
Medical Device Amendments	1976	Created risk-based classification system for medical devices, requiring premarket approval for riskiest (Class III) devices and development of performance standards for less risky products
Drug Price Competition and Patent Term Restoration Act (aka., Hatch-Waxman Amendments)	1984	Incentivized development of generic drugs by allowing the use of Abbreviated New Drug Applications relying on evidence of bioequivalence to pioneer products; authorized exclusivity and patent term extension for pioneer products
Prescription Drug User Fee Act	1992	Authorized the collection of user fees to review New Drug Applications
Medical Device User Fee Amendments	2002	Authorized the collection of user fees to review medical device applications, register establishments, or list marketed products
Generic Drug User Fee Amendments	2012	Authorized the collection of user fees to review Abbreviated New Drug Applications

immunologically based treatments (certain biologics drugs) for psoriasis and other diseases was transferred from the Center for Biologics Evaluation and Research (CBER) to CDER, allowing for a cohesive and more consistent review of those products. Review of vaccines, blood products, tissues, and allergy test products, including patch testing for contact dermatitis remained in CBER. Veterinary dermatology products are regulated by the Center for Veterinary Medicine (CVM). Cosmetics and other personal care products are regulated by the Center for Food Safety and Applied Nutrition (CFSAN)[2,3] Unlike drugs, cosmetic products, and their ingredients, with the exception of color additives, are not required to have premarket approval, though they are subject to regulations related to safety and labeling.

FDA's review of dermatologic products is a collaborative process that draws on the strengths of experts across the agency. Dermatologic products are reviewed by teams within each Center, teams which include experts in all fields relevant for the product, such as dermatologists, other medical specialists, chemists, biologists, pharmacologists, nurses, toxicologists, and engineers, in addition to project managers and individuals with expertise in regulatory law. However, leadership for medical product areas, such as dermatology, can arise at various levels, depending on the product, expertise, and level of oversight needed. Currently, much of the details involved in regulation, like wording for labeling, inspection reports from manufacturing sites, occur at the expert reviewer or team level as guided by institutional guidance, templates, forms, and FDA managers.

Dermatologists have influenced FDA reviews and decision-making over the years by providing the dermatology perspective on risk and benefits of various medical products. This is an important role for any specialist at FDA. There was a high-

Table 2
Board-certified dermatologists who were managers at FDA

Name	Managerial Roles	Years
Dr Clarence Carnot Evans	Dermatology Branch Chief	1987–1992?
Dr Jonathan K. Wilkin	Division Director, DDDDP	1994–2005
Dr Susan Walker	Dermatology Team Leader, DDDDP Division Director, Nutritional Supplements Division Director, DDDDP	1997–2002 2003–2007 2007–2011
Dr Martin Okun	Dermatology Team Leader, DDDDP	1998–2000
Dr Markham C. Luke	Dermatology Team Leader, DDDDP Deputy Office Director, ODE, CDRH Acting Director, Cosmetics Division Director, Therapeutic Performance of Generic Drugs	2001–2008 2008–2016 2012–2013 2016-present
Dr Jill Lindstrom	Dermatology Team Leader, DDDDP Deputy Division Director, DDDDP	2004–2010 2010–2019
RADM Dr Boris Lushniak	Director, Emergency Preparedness (subsequently became Acting Surgeon General for the United States)	2005–2010
Dr Elektra J. Papadopoulos	Associate Office Director, New Drugs and Deputy Director, Clinical Outcomes Assessments	2009-2021

Table 3
Dermatologists who have worked full-time at FDA

Name	FDA Center(s)	Years
Dr Lawrence B. McCaleb	Division of Drugs	1939–1942
Dr Clarence Carnot Evans	Bureau of Medicine CDER	1963–1992?
Dr Phyllis Huene	Bureau of Medicine CDER	1964–2005
Herbert Golomb	Bureau of Medicine	1963-?
Donald Mitchell	Bureau of Medicine	1963-?
Walter Edmundson	Bureau of Medicine	1963-?
Glenn Hays	Bureau of Medicine	c. Late-1960s
Wilson Powell	Bureau of Medicine	c. Late-1960s
John B. Sanders	Bureau of Medicine	c. Late-1960s
Leonard Trilling	Bureau of Medicine	c. Late-1960s
Dr Ramsey Labib	CDER	1990–2002
Dr Ella Toombs	CDER	1989–2002
Dr Brenda Vaughan	CDER	1993–2011
Dr Lois LaGrenade	CDER	1997–2019
Dr Denise Cook	CDER	1995–2022
Dr Jonathan K. Wilkin	CDER	1994–2005
Dr Susan Walker	CDER, CFSAN	1996–2011
Dr Kathy A. O'Connell	CDER, CBER	1996–2014
Dr Martin Okun	CDER	1997–2001
Dr Markham C. Luke	CDER, CDRH, CFSAN	1998-present
Dr Brenda Carr	CDER	2000-present
Dr Elektra Papadopoulos	CBER, CDER	2001-2021
Dr Jill Lindstrom	CDER	2002–2019
Dr Patricia Brown	CDER	2005-present
Dr Jane Leidtka	CDER	2006–2020
Dr Boris Lushniak	OC	2004–2010
Dr Kenneth Katz	CDER	2006–2007
Dr Melinda McCord	CDER	2009-present
Dr Laura Marquart	CDRH	2013-present
Dr Schlomit Halachmi	CDRH	2013-present
Dr Roslyn E. Epps	CDER	2015-present
Dr Melissa Reyes	CDER	2016-present
Dr Felisa Lewis	CDER	2020-present
Dr Mary Kim	CDER	2021-present

level manager at FDA that was often fond of saying that FDA regulates drugs that "treat diseases from heart disease to depression to toenail fungus." Depending on how that statement is interpreted, one could take umbrage on having a certain disease that affects patients one sees and treats for significant concerns and morbidity, at the end of a perceived spectrum. This anecdote speaks to the importance of having adequate representation of a specialty, such as dermatology, at the regulatory conference table, weighed in the balance with other agency experts. As we will discuss, the presence and influence of agency dermatologists is itself an historical development.

The authors have included what they believe is a reasonably complete list of all physicians who were trained and board-certified in dermatology dermatologists who have been part of the FDA. **Table 2** provides a list of board-certified dermatologists who were managers at FDA and the roles they played. **Table 3** offers a list of dermatologists who have worked in various roles across FDA. These lists rely on the authors' knowledge of dermatologists who are or have been working at FDA full-time and may not be fully complete.

ORIGINS OF THE FEDERAL REGULATION OF DERMATOLOGIC PRODUCTS

The 1906 Federal Food and Drugs Act (also known as the Pure Food and Drugs Act) created federal oversight of domestically produced pharmaceuticals for the first time in the United States. The law required drugs to conform to the standards of identity, strength, and purity established by the United States Pharmacopeia and National Formulary and prohibited adulteration or misbranding. The power to enforce this law fell to the US Department of Agriculture's Bureau of Chemistry—renamed the US Food and Drug Administration in 1930—and was largely relegated to regulatory research, postmarket surveillance, product seizures, and criminal prosecution against violative products. However, because the law only applied to foods and drugs, it did not empower the agency to regulate medical devices or cosmetics, which exposed consumers to an increasing number of unsafe and quack products as these industries grew in the early decades of the 20th century.[4]

While the 1906 law empowered the agency to remove violative products from the market, it did not require that products be proven safe or effective before marketing, and it did not authorize the agency to review or approve products before they entered the market. It was precisely for this reason that a toxic antiinfective sulfa drug, Elixir Sulfanilamide, was able to kill more than 100 patients in the fall of 1937—some of whom had

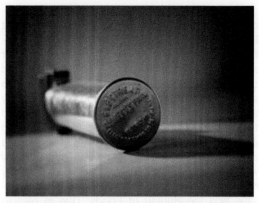

Fig. 2. LashLure and Electreat. *Courtesy* of FDA History Office, Legacy Artifact Collection.

been taking the drug to treat venereal disease. This tragedy laid bare the limitations of the 1906 law and catalyzed the passage of the 1938 Federal Food, Drug, and Cosmetic Act (FFDCA), which not only gave FDA the responsibility for premarket approval of drugs via review of New Drug Applications (NDAs), but also brought cosmetics and medical devices under the agency's authority for the first time.[5] As a testament to the power of these new authorities to protect consumers from fraudulent products, the first legal action that the FDA took under the FFDCA was against Lash Lure, a toxic aniline eyebrow and eyelash dye that blinded several women; one of the first enforcement actions against a medical device was the seizure of the Electreat Mechanical Heart, a transcutaneous electrical nerve stimulation (TENS) device that falsely claimed to treat baldness, acne and aged skin (among dozens of other conditions)[6,7] (**Figs. 1** and **2**).

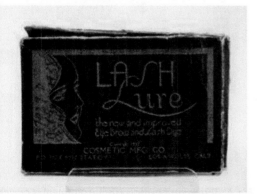

Fig. 1. LashLure and Electreat. *Courtesy of* FDA History Office, Legacy Artifact Collection.

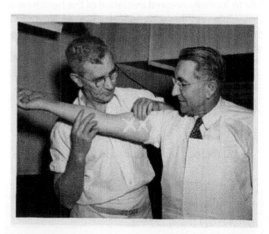

Fig. 3. Draize test. *Courtesy of* FDA History Office, Photograph Collection.

Though FDA hired the agency's first board-certified dermatologist, Lawrence B. McCaleb, at FDA in 1939, dermatology did not truly make landfall at the FDA until the post-World War II era.[8] For several decades thereafter, the regulation of dermatologic medical products was subsumed in various other programs, including pharmacology and toxicology work in the Bureau of Foods and the Bureau of Medicine. By and large, following John Draize's 1944 development of standard dermal and ocular tests of toxicity, the agency was primarily involved in dermal toxicology research that occurred in both the Bureau of Medicine and the Bureau of Foods. Due in part to heightened concerns about carcinogenic food, drug and cosmetic additives that provoked congressional inquiry in the early 1950s, dermal toxicity proved to be a major prong of FDA's regulatory apparatus, which became particularly important in the controversial effort to establish safety parameters for the use of coal tar colors in cosmetics[9] (**Fig. 3**).

Since its original enactment, numerous amendments to the FFDCA have impacted FDA's regulatory authorities. The 1951 Durham-Humphrey Amendments sought to protect patients from misuse of dangerous or habit-forming drugs by making access contingent on the prescription given by a qualified medical professional. Five years after this statutory distinction was made between prescription and over-the-counter (OTC) medicines, 10 pharmaceutical companies petitioned the FDA to convert hydrocortisone ointments from prescription to OTC status. This proposal ignited powerful opposition from the practicing dermatologists concerned about the safety of unrestricted use of these products for skin conditions, which prompted the FDA to hold a public meeting to allow the professional community to formally present evidence of the health risks posed by nonprescription access to cortisone products (eg, the development of Addison's Disease or other endocrinological disorders).[10]

This experience both led the agency to reject the OTC marketing of hydrocortisone ointment (which remained the case until the late-1970s) and actively seek to develop stronger engagement with the American Academy of Dermatology and Syphilology. Irvin Kerlan, Chief of the Bureau of Medicine's Division of Research and Reference, was particularly active in this effort and to develop stronger engagement between the FDA and dermatologists, achieved in part through the formation of an FDA Advisory Committee.[11] By forging this relationship with the professional community, the FDA was better positioned to cultivate dermatologic expertise within the agency in the next decade (**Fig. 4**). This Committee has since been folded into the formal FDA Advisors and Consultants framework (**Box 1**).

DERMATOLOGY MAKES LANDFALL AT THE U.S. FOOD AND DRUG ADMINISTRATION

Over the course of the 1950s, concerns mounted about "me-too" drugs that made overly ambitious claims of efficacy to distinguish themselves from rival products. As a result, the 1962 Drug Amendments required that drugs provide evidence of efficacy in addition to safety before they could be introduced into commerce. The law's efficacy standard created new requirements for the manufacture of dermatologic products and led to action against several wrinkle creams that made unfounded therapeutic claims.[12] But, the law also required the retrospective review of the efficacy of every NDA approved based on safety alone since 1938. Working with the National Academy of Sciences, the FDA arranged for external experts

---

Box 1
Dermatologist chairs of FDA advisory committees

Dermatology, Ophthalmology Drugs Advisory Committee

Dr Lynn A. Drake

Dr William H. Eagelstein

Dr Michael Bigby

Dr Kenneth Katz

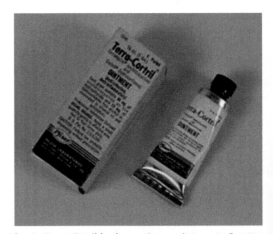

Fig. 4. Terra-Cotril hydrocortisone ointment. *Courtesy of* National Museum of American History, Smithsonian Institution.

to review the approximately 3500 drugs still on the market, which made a total of about 16,000 therapeutic claims. By 1981, this extensive review (known as the Drug Efficacy Study Implementation, or DESI) led to the withdrawal of NDAs for approximately 112 dermatologic products.[13]

DESI addressed prescription drugs, but not the vast number of OTC drugs—which includes a large number of dermatologic drugs. OTC review regulations were promulgated in 1972 requiring retrospective review of all OTC drugs available at the time. The effort relied on the assistance of more than 250 external experts working as special government employees (SGEs), managed by the OTC Drug Division. Each OTC was reviewed by panels of experts, and their review led to the issuance of drug monographs. These monographs describe the active ingredients, what the drug is intended to treat, the dose and route of administration, how the drug will be labeled, and the tests to show that the drug can be considered "generally recognized as safe and effective."[14] OTC monograph drugs that meet the necessary regulatory requirements, including those in the monograph, could be marketed to consumers without FDA review. However, not all OTC drugs are eligible for this process: some nonprescription drug products do require review under an NDA.[15]

In the early 1960s, in accordance with the recommendations of 2 external evaluations by Citizens Advisory Committees, the FDA began large-scale reorganizations and enhanced staffing, in part to support the expansion of regulatory research needs. In 1963, the Bureau of Medicine created a Dermatologic Drugs Group and recruited 4 medical officers specializing in dermatology, assigned to multiple branches in the Bureau of Medicine: Herbert Golomb (Hazardous Substances Branch); Donald Mitchell (Drug Surveillance Branch); Phyllis Huene (Investigational Drug Branch) and Clarence Carnot Evans (Medical Evaluation Branch).[16] Within 5 years, the agency's dermatologic staff had doubled, adding specialists in pharmacology and syphilology, and became mostly consolidated within the Division of Anti-infective Products in the Bureau of Medicine's Office of New Drugs.

For decades thereafter, many FDA dermatologists also maintained clinical practice and/or academic appointments (as was also customary for medical officers specializing in other fields). For instance, throughout much of her nearly 40-year career at FDA, Dr Huene maintained an appointment on the staff of George Washington University Hospital.[17] Others, such as Dr Denise Cook, Admiral Boris Lushniak, Dr Melissa Reyes, and one of the authors (MCL), have treated patients and

taught at the Washington, D.C. Veterans Administration Hospital or at the nation's military hospitals while also working fulltime at the FDA. The ability of FDA dermatologists to interact with experts in the field was a notable asset to regulatory decision making, as the medical products they reviewed became increasingly complex. The agency formalized the role of expert advisors in 1980 with the creation of the Dermatologic Drugs Advisory Committee (renamed the Dermatologic and Ophthalmic Drugs Advisory Committee in 1995).[18]

In the 1970s, the FDA pursued new strategies to ensure the safety of cosmetics by actively engaging the professional community and consumer stakeholders. In 1974, the agency launched a vast study in collaboration with the American Academy of Dermatology to gain information about the nature and scale of injuries caused by cosmetic products. It surveyed nearly 10,000 households, involving approximately 36,000 participants over 3 months. The information gathered led to the 1974 creation of several voluntary compliance programs aimed at strengthening FDA's awareness of adverse events and to enable firms to gain consumer confidence by cooperatively listing their establishments and products with FDA, namely the Voluntary Filing Cosmetic Product Ingredient program and the Voluntary Filing Cosmetic Product Experience Reports program (the Voluntary Cosmetic Product Registry had been established in 1972).[19]

The mid-1970s also ushered in major changes in the regulation of dermatologic devices. The passage of the 1976 Medical Devices Amendments established a risk-based classification system for medical devices, requiring premarket approval of Class III medical devices (eg, implanted devices such as heart valves) and the establishment of performance standards for Class I (low risk, such as syringes) and II devices (requiring special controls, such as electrosurgical devices). Dermatologic devices and surgical products were regulated by the recently established Bureau of Medical Devices and Diagnostic Products until it was reorganized as the Center for Devices and Radiological Health (CDRH) in 1982.[20] Since then, most mainstay dermatologic devices, such as the macroscopic or microscopic visualization and image capture of the skin, automated diagnostic hardware and software, PCR and antibody test kits for infectious diseases, have been reviewed by CDRH before marketing in the United States.[21] However, CBER has regulatory oversight for test kits and materials used to test for allergies, such as allergen patch tests.

The passage of the Medical Device Amendments and the growth of corresponding organizational functions within the agency, put the FDA in a stronger position to regulate innovative dermatologic devices that were developed in the 1980s, including energy-based devices and dermal fillers, which are regulated as implants. Importantly, the legal emphasis on risk evaluation guided the agency's approach to both mitigating and warning consumers about health concerns associated with such products throughout the 1980s and 90s.

EVALUATING AND COMMUNICATING RISKS ASSOCIATED WITH DERMATOLOGIC PRODUCTS

While on one hand, FDA's regulation of dermatologic products has responded to changes in the agency's legal authorities, on the other, therapeutic and diagnostic innovations in the marketplace have strongly impacted FDA's dermatologic products programs. The development of new products has also spurred new considerations and paradigms for interpreting health risks, and FDA has developed new methods for increasing consumer and prescriber awareness of the potential risks associated with specific products. These dynamics were evident in the late-1970s and early-1980s with the emergence of several new products that posed various safety risks.

In the mid-1970s, technology for surgically implanting prosthetic hair fibers in the scalp was first introduced in the US as means of disguising male-pattern baldness. The implants were often made of hundreds of synthetic fibers such as polyester or acrylics, though in some cases were made from chemically processed (not transplanted) human hair. The procedure typically costs thousands of dollars and was not performed by licensed physicians. Predictably, the immune system reacted by rejecting these foreign bodies, causing the implants to fall out or break off, generating infections, scarring, permanent disfiguration, facial swelling, severe pain, and permanent loss of real hair. Between December 1978 and February 1981, the FDA received 166 complaints about adverse reactions caused by these implants (colloquially known as "hair plugs"), and the Federal Trade Commission received an additional 181 complaints. In March 1979, the FDA issued a public warning about the implants and, in June 1983, the agency permanently banned their use—the first medical device to have warranted such a severe action by the FDA.[22,23]

Around the same time, as mounting evidence pointed to a correlation between sun exposure and skin cancer, the FDA contracted with external experts to study commercial sunscreen lotions and present recommendations on ingredients that effectively contribute to Sun Protection Factor (SPF). Because SPF lotions claim therapeutic efficacy, they are considered drugs and require adherence to OTC monograph standards and guidelines, which continue to evolve in accordance with advancements in understanding the impact of ambient ultraviolet (UV) radiation in the development of skin cancer. In 2011, the FDA issued a new sunscreen rule for all OTC sunscreen drug products being marketed without prior FDA review under NDA or Abbreviated NDA (ANDA). The rule required specific labeling elements clarifying the SPF prominently; distinguishing claims that can be made by products with less than SPF 15 from claims made by products with SPF 15 or higher (the latter can claim "if used as directed with other sun protection measures (see Directions), decreases the risk of skin cancer and early skin aging caused by the sun"); standardizing requirements for testing to support labeling of "broad spectrum" and duration of water resistance; and requiring specific information on how to apply and on risks of sun exposure.[24]

While FDA-regulated SPF products provided some protection against UV light, the agency was also mandated to set performance standards for UV radiation devices, including indoor tanning beds (classified as "sunlamp products"). In the fall of 1987, FDA issued regulations requiring that all tanning beds be equipped with timers and labeled with clear directions for use, including instructions that users wear protectant goggles to protect their eyes to prevent injury.[25,26] Slightly over 3 decades later, mounting evidence linking UV radiation with melanoma prompted FDA to convene an Advisory Committee meeting on the safety of these products in 2010, and in 2014 to reclassify sunlamp products from Class I to Class II medical devices, making them subject to 510K premarket notification, quality system regulation, labeling requirements, and medical device adverse event reporting. In addition, the agency required all indoor tanning devices to bear a boxed warning stating that children under 18 should not use such devices.[27]

The early 1980s also saw major innovation in treating aging and scarred skin: the use of silicone dermal fillers to reduce wrinkles and acne scars. Though medical-grade injectable silicone oil—a gel-like form of siloxane used in lubricants and caulk—had been used since the 1960s as a topical product to prevent skin maceration and as an implant for breast augmentation, the subdermal injection of this product presented a new regulatory challenge for FDA. Injectable silicone, when applied to change the structure of the body, is a medical device. Therefore, under the 1976 Medical Device Amendments, the FDA is responsible for determining the safety of injectable sterile silicone, which has been found to cause a range of side effects from skin discoloration to the formation of cysts, tumors, and cardiovascular blockages due to the migration of silicone to other organs, including the lungs and the brain.[28]

Concerned by the documented adverse events associated with silicone fillers, FDA developed a testing program that would be carried out by a panel of physicians and restrict its use to severe facial deformities, with several years follow-up.[29] The original manufacturer eventually suspended efforts to market the silicone. However, silicone injections continued, not always in the hands of licensed providers. In 2017, in response to reports of body contouring procedures and facial filler procedures with silicone, FDA issued a stark safety communication, outlining the risks of infections, permanent disfigurement, embolism, stroke, and death.[30] The safety communication is an example of FDA's use of press releases and educational materials to promote broad public awareness of risks.

An even more apropos example of the ways in which FDA regulation has shaped and been shaped by new dermatologic products began with the first approval of isotretinoin (marketed under the brand name Accutane) for the treatment of cystic acne in 1982. Before the drug's approval, animal studies detected teratogenic effects, so it was introduced to the market with explicit warning that it should not be used by pregnant women. In 1984, this warning was enhanced with a requirement that the products include a recommendation that patients take a pregnancy test before beginning treatment with isotretinoin. These strategies were not sufficient to prevent an estimated 1300 babies from being born with isotretinoin-induced birth defects by the end of 1986.[31] FDA's Dermatologic Drugs Advisory Committee recommended specific labeling changes targeted to both patients and practitioners, and the agency worked with the manufacturer to develop strategies to more impactfully educate patients about the potential risks, including extensive pregnancy prevention materials. In 2005, the FDA launched the iPLEDGE program to use telecommunications systems to communicate risk information to both patients and doctors and enhance ethics compliance.[32] (Fig. 5)

Concerns about Accutane risk mitigation overlapped with the FDA's review of an application for the use of thalidomide to treat Erythema nodosum leprosum caused by Hansen's Disease and multiple myeloma. Since first being linked with

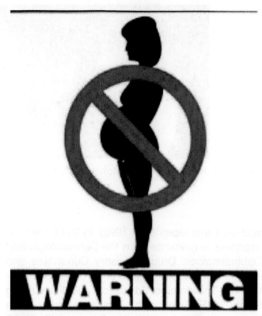

Fig. 5. Accutane warning. *Courtesy of* FDA History Office Still Image Collections.

severe birth defects in 1961, thalidomide had been banned in the US, and had prompted FDA's 1977 recommendation that women of child-bearing potential be excluded from clinical trials out of an abundance of precaution (this

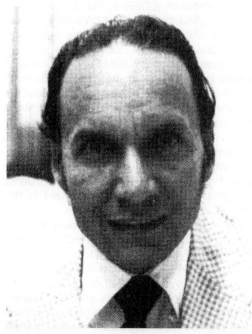

Fig. 6. Clarence Carnot Evans. *Courtesy of* FDA History Office Still Image Collections.

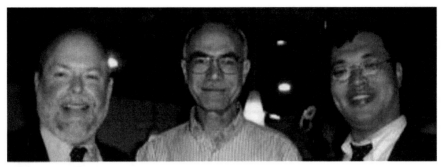

Fig. 7. Drs. Jonathan Wilkin, Mohamed Al'Osh and Markham Luke.

guidance was repealed in 1992). In 1998, the FDA appealed to guidance from the Dermatologic and Ophthalmologic Drugs Advisory Committee and worked with the manufacturer to develop a System for Thalidomide Education and Prescribing Safety (STEPS) program, which in many ways became a pilot for both the Accutane iPLEDGE program and the development of Risk Evaluation and Mitigation Strategies (REMS) programs authorized by the Food and Drug Administration Amendments Act of 2007.[33]

REGULATORY CHALLENGES AND THERAPEUTIC INNOVATIONS IN THE 21ST CENTURY

The establishment of the Center for Drug Evaluation and Research (CDER) in 1987 entailed large-scale reorganization of the FDA's drug review, research, and compliance functions that led to organizational changes for the Dermatologic Drugs Branch. Clarence Carnot Evans, an original member (and long-time team lead) of the Dermatologic Drugs Group was named Branch Chief. Over the next half dozen years, the dermatologic drugs program continued to grow in size and significance, and, in 1997, merged with dental drug products and elevated to the division level. Jonathan Wilkin was named director of the newly created Division of Dermatologic and Dental Drug Products (DDDDP) and continued in that role until 2005.[34] (**Figs. 6** and **7**).

One of the more significant developments for dermatologists at FDA in the new millennium was the advent of aesthetic dermatologic products. This terminology was generated at FDA by the emergence of a new class of drugs and devices intended to use medical means, such as therapeutics or surgery to enhance one's physical appearance (with no other significant medical benefit, with the exception of possible improvements in mental health). The term "aesthetic" was preferred

by FDA regulators of drugs, biologics, and devices, to differentiate these from "cosmetics" which were regulated in CFSAN. FDA discouraged off-label promotion of drugs like botulinum toxin and tretinoin for aesthetic conditions, requiring manufacturers to study those drugs for the indications for which they were promoted.[35]

A good example is the approval of topical tretinoin, a drug originally marketed for the treatment of acne, for aesthetic purposes. For years before the approval of an aesthetic formulation for tretinoin in 1995, the manufacturer of the drug had been promoting the off-label use of its acne drug for treating fine wrinkles through dermatologists and the media. The FDA approved labeling (August, 2000) for the tretinoin 0.02% product was ground-breaking in that it was one of the first products to use a Patient-Reported Outcome (PRO) and reported in labeling as a measure of its effectiveness.[36] The labeling described "Patient Self-Assessments" of fine wrinkling and other aesthetic endpoints. PRO instruments have

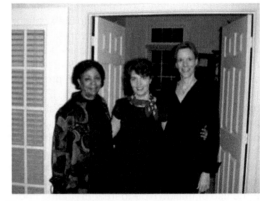

Fig. 8. Drs. Brenda Vaughan, Elektra Papadopoulos, and Jill Lindstrom.

become an important part of other drugs, including those for indications other than in dermatology (**Fig. 8**).

One of the most conspicuous icons of aesthetic medicine is the use of botulinum toxins for wrinkles. In 2000, the FDA issued the first such product approval for botulinum toxin "for the temporary improvement of appearance of 62 glabellar lines," sparking a popular trend in Botox injections.[37]

Though the authority to regulate biological products was transferred to FDA in 1972 when the Bureau of Biologics was moved from the National Institutes of Health and reorganized under the FDA, for the duration of the 20th century there were few advancements in the dermatologic application of biologics. However, since 2000, dermatologic product regulation at FDA has seen the rise of therapeutic biologics for the treatment of certain skin conditions that are thought to be immune-mediated, that is, psoriasis and atopic dermatitis. In 2009, FDA approved the first monoclonal antibody for a dermatologic purpose, approving the use of ustekinumab for the treatment of plaque psoriasis, charting the course for a wide array of biological therapies for psoriasis and other inflammatory disorders. More recently, in March 2017, FDA approved the first biological product, dupilumab, for the treatment of atopic dermatitis.[38]

As we enter the third decade of the 21st century, FDA pharmacologists working together with other regulators, including our dermatologists, advanced major breakthroughs in the regulation of generic dermatologic drugs by developing a viable in vitro approach to topical drug bioequivalence for generic drug approvals. This was achieved through a multi-year research program that studied gels, ointments, lotion, and cream products containing a number of active drugs (eg, acyclovir, metronidazole, nystatin, triamcinolone acetonide, lidocaine, prilocaine, and diclofenac), establishing tailored product-specific approaches for many topical products. As a result of this program, it is hopeful that the pharmaceutical industry will be able to develop generic equivalents of many high-cost dermatologic drugs, vastly reducing medical costs to patients.[39]

Today, other advances continue to be made in the science of dermatopharmacology and the evaluation of effectiveness of treatments used for dermatologic disease, spearheaded by investments made by FDA in studying clinical outcomes, new methods to analyze drugs in the skin, and new methods to incorporate artificial intelligence, data analysis, and pharmacokinetic/pharmacodynamic modeling into the science of the treatment of skin diseases.

CLINICS CARE POINTS

- The history of dermatology and the tools used for treatment and diagnosis by dermatologists are intertwined with the history of product regulation at the Food and Drug Administration.
- Many dermatologists at FDA have played an important role in shaping the landscape of treatments and diagnostics over the years.
- FDA regulation of dermatologic products involves a mix of legal, scienfic, and risk comprehension.

ACKNOWLEDGMENTS

The authors would like to acknowledge Susan Levine, JD, Deputy Director in FDA's Division of Public Policy in the Office of Generic Drugs, and Barbara Kass, FDA Writer/Editor for a critical and careful read-thru of our article.

REFERENCES

1. FDA At A Glance. Nov. 2020. Available at: https://www.fda.gov/media/143704/download. Accessed August 5, 2021.
2. Available at: https://www.fda.gov/cosmetics. Accessed June 8, 2022.
3. United States Code, Title 21, Chapter 9, Subchapter II, section 321.2(i).
4. Janssen W. The Story of the Law Behind the Labels. FDA Consumer June 1981. Available at: https://www.fda.gov/media/116890/download. Accessed August 5, 2021.
5. Young JH. Sulfanilamide and Diethylene Glycol. In: Parascondola J, Wharton JC, editors. Chemistry and modern society: historical essays in honor of Aaron J. Ihde. Washington D.C: American Chemical Society; 1983. p. 105–25.
6. Adulteration of Lash Lure. U. S. v. 23 Boxes of Lash Lure (and 38 other seizure actions against the same product). Default decrees of condemnation and destruction. 1940. Case number 1. Available at: https://fdanj.nlm.nih.gov/catalog/csnj00001. Accessed August 5, 2021.
7. Misbranding of Electreat Mechanical Heart. U. S. v.6 Electreat Mechanical Hearts. Tried to the court. Judgment for the Government. Decree of condemnation and destruction. Case number 376. Available at: https://fdanj.nlm.nih.gov/catalog/ddnj00376. Accessed August 5, 2021.

8. McCaleb Appointed to Drug Division. Food and Drug Review 1940;37.

9. Importance of Hair Dye Patch Test Stressed. Food and Drug Review 1944:154.

10. U.S. Food and Drug Administration. Press Release. Mar. 31, 1956.

11. Food and Drug Review 1951:191.

12. U.S. Food and Drug Administration. Press Release. May 15, 1964.

13. U.S. Food and Drug Administration. Annual Report. 1980-1982.

14. Over-the-Counter (OTC) Drug Monograph Process. Available at: https://www.fda.gov/drugs/over-counter-otc-drug-monograph-process. Accessed May 4, 2021.

15. Over-the-Counter (OTC) | nonprescription drugs. Available at: https://www.fda.gov/drugs/how-drugs-are-developed-and-approved/over-counter-otc-non prescription-drugs. Accessed May 4, 2021.

16. FDA Personnel Rosters, 1961, 1965, 1967 and 1969. FDA History Office research files. Silver Spring, MD.

17. United States Congress. House of Representatives, Committee on Government Operations. Drug Safety: Hearings Before a Subcommittee of the Committee on Government Operations, Eighty-eighth Congress, Second Session, Parts 1-5, March 24, 25, April 8, and June 3, 1964 . Washington, D.C. U.S. Government Printing Office, 1964:915.

18. U.S. Department of Health and Human Services, Food and Drug Administration. Advisory Committees; Establishment. Final Rule. Federal Register Nov. 28, 1980; 45: 79026.

19. U.S. Food and Drug Administration. Press Release. Sept. 11, 1974 and Jun. 29, 1975.

20. CDRH Milestones. Available at: https://www.fda.gov/media/108643/download. Accessed August 5, 2021.

21. Dang JM, Krause D, Felten RP, et al. Medical device regulation: what a practicing dermatologist should know. Dermatol Ther 2009;22(3):241–5. Erratum in: Dermatol Ther. 2009 Jul-Aug;22(4):395. Luke, Markham K [corrected to Luke, Markham C]. PMID: 19453348.

22. U.S. Food and Drug Administration. Press Release. June 3, 1983.

23. Hair Fibers Banned. FDA Consumer 1983; September:26-7.

24. U.S. Food and Drug Administration. Guidance for Industry. Labeling and effectiveness testing: sunscreen drug products for over-the counter human use – small entity compliance guide. 2012. Available at: https://www.fda.gov/files/drugs/published/Labeling-and-Effectiveness-Testing–Sunscreen-Drug-Products-for-Over-The-Counter-Human-Use-%E2%80%94-Small-Entity-Compliance-Guide_pdf.pdf. Accessed August 5, 2021.

25. Farley D. Laser treatment to go: outpatient use of healing light abound. FDA Consumer 1987:22-28.

26. Hopkins H. Tan now pay later. FDA Consumer. 1982: 9–11.

27. U.S. Food and Drug Administration. Press Release. May 29, 2014.

28. Klevan P. New face lift not all smiles. FDA Consumer 1979:15.

29. Goulian D Jr. Current status of liquid injectable silicone. Aesthetic Plast Surg 1978;2(1):247–50.

30. FDA warns against use of injectable silicone for body contouring and enhancement: FDA Safety Communication. 2017. Available at: www.fda.gov/medical-devices/safety-communications/fda-warns-against-use-injectable-silicone-body-contouring-and-enhancement-fda-safety-communication. Accessed April 6, 2021.

31. Sun M. Anti-acne drug poses dilemma for FDA. Science 1988;240:714–5.

32. U.S. Food and Drug Administration. FDA announces strengthened risk management program to enhance safe use of isotretinoin (Accutane) for treating severe acne. August 12, 2004. Available at: https://web.archive.org/web/20060216205546/http://www.fda.gov/bbs/topics/NEWS/2005/NEW01218.html. Accessed June 8, 2022.

33. Zeldis JB, Williams BA, Thomas SD, et al. A comprehensive program for controlling and monitoring access to thalidomide. Clin Ther 1999;21(2):319–30.

34. The role of DDDP Division Director is currently filled by Dr. Kendall A. Marcus, who is board-certified in Infectious Disease, and was filled by Dr. Stanka Kukich, an internist, from 2006-2007.

35. Lupo M. Tox outside the box: off-label aesthetic uses of botulinum toxin. J Drugs Dermatol 2016;15:9.

36. Renova (tretinoin) Drug Approval Package. NDA #021108. Available at: https://www.accessdata.fda.gov/drugsatfda_docs/nda/2000/21-108_Renova.cfm. Accessed June 8, 2022.

37. U.S. Food and Drug Administration. Guidance for Industry. Upper facial lines: developing botulinum toxin drug products. Available at: https://www.fda.gov/files/drugs/published/Upper-Facial-Lines—Developing-Botulinum-Toxin-Drug-Products.pdf. Accessed June 8, 2022.

38. U.S. Food and Drug Administration. Press Release. March 28, 2017. Available at: Available at: https://www.fda.gov/news-events/press-announcements/fdaapproves-new-eczema-drug-dupixent. Accessed June 8, 2022.

39. Raney S. Bioequivalence of complex topical generics: in vitro and in vivo" FDA grand rounds webcast October 8, 2020. Available at: https://www.fda.gov/news-events/fda-meetings-conferences-and-workshops/bioequivalence-complex-topical-generics-vitro-and-vivo-10082020-10082020#event-information. Accessed June 8, 2022.

The Food and Drug Administration's Role in Dermatologic Drug Development

Felisa S. Lewis, MD, MPH*, Kendall A. Marcus, MD

KEYWORDS

- Dermatology • Drug development • Food and Drug Administration • Investigational New Drug
- New Drug Application

KEY POINTS

- The mission of the Food and Drug Administration (FDA) is to ensure the safety and effectiveness of dermatologic drugs, as authorized by the Federal Food, Drug, and Cosmetic Act (FD&CA) and regulated by Title 21, Code of Federal Regulations (CFR).
- Unlike federal regulations, FDA guidance for industry reflect the Agency's current thinking on a topic and are not legally binding on drug sponsors or the FDA.
- Because drug development is continually evolving, the Division of Dermatology and Dentistry (DDD) in the Center of Drug Evaluation and Research (CDER) actively encourages dermatologic drug development by regularly engaging with sponsors and other stakeholders.
- The primary basis for FDA approval of a drug marketing application is the benefit-risk assessment.

INTRODUCTION

The process of discovering and bringing any new molecular entity (NME) to market is one that requires persistence, significant financial resources, and a broad horizon. Although pharmaceutical companies may carry the immediate burden of investing money and time, there are other major stakeholders in drug development including the Food and Drug Administration (FDA), researchers, patients, prescribers, and payers. Each group has obligations, priorities, and influences that shape their behavior (**Table 1**).

These relationships are complex. There is an inherent tension when the FDA and pharmaceutical companies, the stakeholders most actively involved in drug development, have different perspectives and motivations, which can result in competing messages to researchers, patients, patient advocacy organizations, prescribers, and payers. These stakeholders have their own agendas and perceptions and seek to influence the FDA and pharmaceutical industry. Nonetheless, all share a common goal—delivering safe and effective drugs to dermatologic patients.

Certain factors influence stakeholder decisions about the development of dermatologic drugs (**Box 1**). The first two, scientific understanding of the pathophysiology of dermatologic conditions and genomic sequencing and its application to dermatologic conditions, significantly influence researchers and pharmaceutical companies in the

Authors' Note: While the authors are employees of the US Food and Drug Administration, the opinions and views expressed in this article are their own and do not reflect US Food and Drug Administration policy or official guidance.

Division of Dermatology and Dentistry, Office of Inflammation and Immunology, Office of New Drugs, Center for Drug Evaluation and Research, Food and Drug Administration, WO22, 10903 New Hampshire Avenue, Silver Spring, MD 20993-0002, USA

* Corresponding author.

E-mail address: felisa.lewis@fda.hhs.gov

Dermatol Clin 40 (2022) 249–263
https://doi.org/10.1016/j.det.2022.02.001
0733-8635/22/Published by Elsevier Inc.

Abbreviations	
IND	Investigational New Drug
NDA	New Drug Application
BLA	Biologic License Application
FDA	Food and Drug Administration
CDER	Center for Drug Evaluation and Research
DDD	Division of Dermatology and Dentistry
NME	new molecular entity
GCP	good clinical practice
FD&CA	Food, Drug, and Cosmetic Act
CFR	Code of Federal Regulation
PDUFA	Prescription Drug User Fee Act
PREA	Pediatric Research Equity Act
REMS	Risk Evaluation and Mitigation Strategy
MUsT	maximal usage trial
PK	pharmokinetic
PMR	postmarketing requirement
PMC	postmarketing commitment
BSA	body surface area
CMC	chemistry, manufacturing, and controls
USC	United States Code
BRA	benefit-risk assessment
EOP2	End-of-Phase 2

process of drug discovery. "Medical necessity," a payer term that originated in the 1940s with private insurance and adopted by Medicare and Medicaid, was borne out of a need to justify insurance coverage, but was largely left to a physician's discretion as to what patient care was "appropriate and effective" to diagnose and treat a medical condition.[19] As the cost of health care and patient demands increased, administrators introduced "cost-effectiveness" as a value-based consideration for coverage in the 1970s, requiring comparisons of "necessity" between medical conditions and treatments. The Social Security Act defined "medical necessity" for Medicare in terms of morbidity and mortality and excluding what was "not reasonable and necessary for the diagnosis or treatment of illness or injury or to improve the functioning of a malformed body member."[20] As a result, population-level practice standards superseded professional medical judgment of individual physicians (and the patient) in the determination of necessity for patient care. A likely unintended consequence of this approach was the creation of a hierarchy of medical needs that established dermatologic conditions as relatively benign since the most common dermatologic conditions do not result directly in death or chronic and progressive physical dysfunction. In addition, because the most familiar dermatologic conditions may seem

to improve over time or patients do not seek medical care, the number of affected dermatologic patients is frequently underestimated. The effect has been to minimize the importance of treatment of dermatologic conditions, stunting the development of most dermatologic drugs,[21] with the notable exception of those used to treat metastatic melanoma. Lastly, one of the primary challenges affecting the design of clinical trials of dermatologic drugs has been the lack of efficacy endpoints that adequately and reliably assess subjective aspects (such as itch or pain) of a dermatologic condition that may provide a clinically meaningful benefit to a patient, even without objective improvement of their skin disease.

Despite the complexities and challenges in this environment, the FDA approved 46 NMEs for dermatologic indications from 2011 to 2022, 27 of these within the Division of Dermatology and Dentistry (DDD), the division in the CDER responsible for regulating dermatologic drugs in development and seeking approval for marketing (Appendix 1). Among these are apremilast (2014), a novel oral therapy for psoriatic arthritis and psoriasis; clascoterone cream 1% (2020), a first-in-class treatment of acne; and afamelanotide (2019), the first FDA-approved drug to increase pain-free light exposure in patients with the rare disease erythropoietic protoporphyria (EPP).

Table 1
Key stakeholders in drug development

Stakeholder	Obligations	Priorities	Influences
FDA[1,2] (CDER and DDD)	Ensuring that approved drugs are safe and effective	Favorable drug benefit-risk assessment supported by scientific rigor Drug quality Patient and prescriber education	Public perception Communication of benefit vs risk Federal funding
Pharmaceutical companies[3–5]	Profit for investors	Market size (number of patients affected) Market exclusivity Trial efficiency Probability of success Return on investment	Research & development costs Risk tolerance of investors Regulation (FDA and environmental) Market competition Formulary tiers Public perception
Researchers (including academia and scientists)[6–8]	Advance scientific understanding of dermatologic disease	Discovery of target to solve medical problem Characterization of target molecule	Scientific and technological advances Financial resources Patient advocacy organizations Employer priorities Personal research interests
Prescribers[8–10]	Providing optimal care for their patients	Drug safety and effectiveness Drug access/availability Identifying gaps/medical need	FDA approval of drugs Drug/health literacy Time constraints Clinical guidelines Formularies Pharmaceutical reps Patient demands
Patients[11–14]	Define clinically meaningful impacts	Drug safety and effectiveness Quality of life	Drug/health literacy Prescriber decisions Competing "experts" Direct-to-consumer advertising Drug access/cost Insurance coverage
Patient advocacy organizations (PAOs)[15–17]	Engage with decision-makers on behalf of patients with dermatologic conditions	Increase funding for disease research and treatment Educate and support patients and public Greater visibility for constituents	Donors (often pharma) Researchers
Payors (public)[18]	Efficient budget management	Size of budget relative to population supported	Cost of health care Determinations of medical necessity Competing government budget priorities
Payors (private)[13]	Profit for investors	Favorable drug benefit-cost assessment	Cost of health care Determinations of medical necessity Optimizing beneficiary mix

Abbreviations: CDER, Center for Drug Evaluation and Research; DDD, Division of Dermatology and Dentistry; FDA, Food and Drug Administration.

> **Box 1**
> **Factors influencing decisions about dermatologic drug development**
>
> Scientific understanding of pathophysiology of dermatologic conditions
>
> Genomic sequencing and its application to dermatologic conditions
>
> Considerations of dermatologic conditions as "medical" vs "cosmetic"
>
> Perceptions about "seriousness" of dermatologic conditions relative to other medical conditions (such as cancer)
>
> Size of patient population affected by dermatologic conditions compared with other medical conditions (such as heart disease or diabetes)
>
> Availability of instruments to measure clinically meaningful but subjective components of a dermatologic condition in an objective and consistent method to demonstrate effectiveness

CDER continues to support expanding the availability of drugs to treat rare diseases through the Rare Diseases Program[22] and incorporating patient perspectives through the "Patient-Focused Drug Development"[23] initiative in accordance with the 21st Century Cures Act and the FDA Reauthorization Act of 2017. Forums for gathering input from stakeholders have included FDA-led meetings (e.g., for alopecia areata in 2017[24]) and patient listening sessions (eg, a patient-led session on Gorlin Syndrome[25]).

Within the context of the regulatory framework that governs the interactions of DDD and the pharmaceutical companies who sponsor investigational drugs during the drug development process, we will discuss how the FDA's policies and practices have continued to evolve to incorporate scientific advances and to facilitate approval for drugs in a timely manner for a broad spectrum of patients. We will provide several examples to highlight areas where DDD found common ground with stakeholders to increase the therapeutic options for dermatologic patients while still maintaining regulatory standards required for approval.

THE REGULATORY FRAMEWORK

The 1962 Kefauver-Harris Drug Amendments of the Federal Food, Drug, and Cosmetic Act (FD&CA)[26] provides the legal basis for the FDA mandate to ensure "the safety, effectiveness, and reliability of drugs."[27] The strategic framework for new drug development and approval is further outlined by regulation in Title 21 section 355 of the US Code (USC)[28] and sections 312 and 314 of the Code of Federal Regulations (CFR).[29] These regulations delineate the distinct roles of the sponsor and the FDA. The sponsor is primarily responsible for "managing the overall development of their drugs…, determining the nature and timing of regulatory submissions…, soliciting input and guidance from the FDA…, and providing well-organized and complete…submissions…to the FDA for review."[30] Meanwhile, the FDA must ensure the safety and rights of subjects at all phases of development; during Phases 2 and 3, "ensure that the quality of the scientific evaluation…is adequate to permit the evaluation of the drug's effectiveness and safety"[31]; enforce good clinical practice (GCP) and human subject protections (HSP) requirements; review submissions; and take regulatory actions as necessary.

A drug or biologic that is being studied in human subjects is known as an Investigational New Drug (IND). When the sponsor of the drug believes there is sufficient evidence for approval, the company submits a New Drug Application (NDA) for drugs or Biologic License Application (BLA) for biologics[1] with the goal of obtaining approval to market the product in the USA. From the FDA perspective, drug development can be broken down into four stages: *pre-IND, IND, NDA/BLA,* and *postmarketing.*

The general process and requirements for the different phases of drug development are outlined in 21 CFR 312.21,[32] although there is room for operational interpretation by the FDA. Broadly, the FDA communicates their interpretation and current thinking on topics that apply across the Agency in the form of Guidances for Industry.[33] Individual guidances, which may be updated as science and technology evolve around drug development, provide sponsors more specific details about the FDA's current intent and expectations to ensure standards are met, with the goal of a more consistent and transparent review and approval process. To be clear though, unlike the requirements set out in regulations, guidances are not legally binding on sponsors *or* the FDA. Guidances serve as "rules of the road" but the development process for each molecular entity will be unique.

---

[1]For the purposes of this article, biologics (generally defined as large complex molecules produced through biotechnology in a living system) follow a similar process as drugs (small chemically-synthesized molecules) in DDD.

For this reason, there are formal meeting opportunities available during the review and approval process for a sponsor to engage and communicate with DDD. The purpose and structure of these meetings are laid out in Prescription Drug User Fee Act (PDUFA) V and 21 CFR 312.47,[34] with more detail provided in the FDA documents listed in Appendix 2. These meetings are highly recommended because they are beneficial for both the sponsor and DDD, but they are not mandatory and should be initiated/requested by the sponsor. Formal meetings allow for greater transparency between the sponsor and DDD about the development program of a specific drug; however, they are purposefully narrow in focus. Before the meeting, sponsors submit background materials and specific questions about the structural aspects of the program for which they are seeking feedback and/or agreement from the FDA. For example, if a sponsor wishes to deviate from the generally accepted guidance documents or has developed a novel trial design, a meeting is the ideal opportunity to introduce and discuss these proposals with DDD.

In the sections about the drug development stages that follow, we'll first review the regulatory requirements and discuss the recommended formal meeting(s) with FDA. The list of the most applicable FDA guidances for that stage of drug development is available in Appendix 2. Finally, we'll provide an example of a recently-approved dermatologic drug reviewed in DDD that used a process or guidance to facilitate the progress at that stage of the drug's development program.

Pre-Investigational New Drug Stage

Regulation

It is well-known that pharmaceutical companies invest significant resources to discover new molecular entities (NME) that have the potential to treat human diseases. Before testing drugs in humans, pharmaceutical companies must first establish the properties of an NME (also known as characterization), as well as conduct multiple nonclinical pharmacology and toxicology tests (**Box 2**) to establish baseline knowledge about its potential for toxicity in humans. The results of these tests are used to estimate a safe first-in-human (FIH) starting and maximum exploratory doses, identify organ targets and adverse effects to establish safety monitoring

---

Box 2
Typical nonclinical tests conducted in the pre-IND/early IND stage for dermatology drugs[35]

Pharmacokinetics (absorption, distribution, metabolism, and excretion, ADME)

Pharmacodynamics (mechanism(s) of action)

Acute, subacute, and chronic toxicity (single- and repeat-dose)

Determination of first-in-human dose and no observed adverse effect level (NOAEL)

Genotoxicity

Reproduction toxicity

Developmental toxicity

Carcinogenicity

Local tolerance studies

Immunotoxicity

Photosafety

---

requirements, and predict risk for special populations (pregnancy, pediatrics), among others.

When the sponsor determines that the drug has been sufficiently characterized and demonstrated potential to treat a particular condition based on these tests, the sponsor can seek feedback from the FDA about their development program during a pre-IND meeting. Issues that might be covered during this meeting include safety issues related to the proper identification, strength, quality, purity, or potency of the investigational drug[36]; animal studies conducted to support human testing; preliminary evaluation of a Phase 1 trial design; and adequacy of the preclinical program to support the initiation of an IND.[37]

DDD and dermal safety studies

Because a number of dermatologic drugs are applied topically, dermal safety studies have been traditionally initiated during the pre-IND phase in animal models and then later in healthy human volunteers[2] to evaluate for local skin reactions such as irritation, contact sensitization, phototoxicity, and photoallergenicity at the site of application. However, there have been concerns about the limitations and the broad applicability of these tests to actual clinical use. For example, dermal safety studies in animals can be complicated by grooming habits that result in the

---

[2]Dermal safety studies are done later when the final to-be-marketed formulation has been determined. In early clinical development, human studies on dermal safety may be done for selection of vehicle or strength of the active ingredient.

ingestion of the drug and increased toxicity or restrictive banding to keep patches in place causing hepatonecrosis.[38] Dermal safety evaluations in humans in the early stages of development are performed on the normal skin of healthy subjects (not on lesional skin of patients) and under occlusion (applied as a patch), conditions not reflective of real-life use for topical drug products. There are also ethical concerns about induction and potential permanence of unnecessary contact sensitization. Generally, the results of these tests haven't been incorporated into the labeling of topical drug products.

Review of data accumulated over years with this approach indicated that results generated from these human dermal safety studies provide information on the potential of the topical drug product to elicit each relevant dermal toxicity but may not accurately convey the actual risk from clinical use. DDD convened a public workshop of FDA scientists along with representatives from the pharmaceutical industry and other stakeholders in September 2018 to discuss these concerns.[39] The consensus that certain dedicated dermal safety studies may not be necessary across the board if the assessment is conducted during Phase 3 trials led to a draft guidance, *Contact Dermatitis from Topical Drug Products for Cutaneous Application: Human Safety Assessment*.[40]

DDD's activities coincided with a larger FDA effort to support and incorporate advances in science and technology, broadly called new approach methodologies (NAMs), during nonclinical drug development.[41] Led by CDER toxicologists, the FDA produced a Predictive Toxicology Roadmap[42] and formed the Alternative Methods Working Group,[43] to identify, introduce, and test NAMs that could ultimately replace animal models. With the application of pharmacogenomics and proteomics, the goal is that NAMs using in vitro, in chemico, and in silico testing, will be shown to be more predictive of human toxicities and outcomes and improve regulatory efficiency. For pharmaceutical companies, such testing strategies have the potential to enhance drug discovery and expedite drug development. If a sponsor is considering using a NAM to derive or supplement nonclinical data to support clinical studies, the pre-IND meeting is an ideal forum to provide DDD details about the methodology, demonstrate that it is appropriate for use, and gain FDA feedback on its acceptability.

Investigational New Drug Stage

Regulation

Investigational new drugs can only be tested in humans in clinical trials in the United States under an IND. An NME will go through the traditional pathway which consists of a sequence of three increasingly stringent phases: Phase 1, FIH studies, often conducted with a small number of healthy subjects to gather information about pharmacokinetics, toxicities, adverse events, and dosing; Phase 2 proof-of-concept efficacy studies and dose-finding studies in affected subjects; and Phase 3 studies with larger numbers of affected subjects to confirm the efficacy and further describe the safety profile of the drug. With some drugs, a company may choose to conduct Phase 1 or 2 studies outside of the United States.[44] A key milestone meeting during the IND stage is the End-of-Phase 2 (EOP2) meeting.[3] Some topics for consideration are the Phase 3 trial design(s) including dose selection, endpoint selection, and the number of subjects needed to provide an adequate efficacy and safety database; pediatric studies, including those required under the Pediatric Research Equity Act (PREA); the adequacy of the supporting nonclinical and clinical pharmacology data; and any additional information needed to support an NDA/BLA submission.[37] A Type C development meeting is appropriate for requesting feedback on other aspects of development and can be requested at any stage of IND development.

Maximal usage studies for topical products

A common strategy for treating dermatologic conditions is the use of topical products. There are multiple advantages to topical therapy compared with drugs taken orally or administered by injection. The primary advantage is that the drug is directly delivered to the target area (avoiding first-pass metabolism), and with the goal to produce less systemic exposure. Thus, topical application decreases the possibility of drug–drug interaction and potential toxicity to other organs. Several factors intrinsic to the patient and disease can impact topical drug absorption to the degree that systemic exposure (and increased risk of off-target adverse reactions) becomes a concern. The possibility of systemic absorption increases when the topical drug is applied to thin-skinned areas (eg, face or intertriginous areas) or the skin barrier is compromised due to the pathophysiology of the disease (eg, a psoriatic plaque) or symptoms (eg, intense pruritus leading to

---

[3]For drugs that are in expedited review programs, this meeting may take place at the End of Phase 1.

scratching). Other variables that increase the risk of systemic absorption include application to larger body surface area and increased frequency and/or duration of application. For pediatric and geriatric populations, there are additional factors to consider. Neonates and infants have a higher rate of percutaneous absorption due to a larger ratio of total body surface area (BSA) to body mass compared with adults, greater perfusion in the subcutaneous layer, and more immature drug-metabolizing structures.[45] Skin atrophy occurs with aging and excessive lifetime sun exposure, putting geriatric patients at increased risk for systemic adverse reactions, which can be compounded if the patient also has decreased organ function, takes other systemic medications, or has significant comorbidities.[46] The most familiar example of this phenomenon is the development of hypothalamic–pituitary–adrenal (HPA) axis suppression with topical corticosteroid use, with the greatest potential occurring in infants due to their high ratio of total BSA to body mass.[47]

To characterize the greatest degree of systemic absorption for a topical drug, a sponsor will typically conduct a maximal usage trial (MUsT, also known as a maximal use pharmokinetic trial) during the IND stage after the expected dosing regimen for the drug's indication has been selected, typically during Phase 2 trials. With the expectation that the highest risk of systemic absorption will occur when a patient applies the maximal amount prescribed according to the proposed labeling, the parameters of a MUsT design are required to reflect the conditions in which maximal application is anticipated, including the total amount of affected BSA treated in a single application, with the application of the highest proposed strength at the maximum anticipated frequency, and for a duration sufficient to achieve maximal drug absorption. In addition, the MUsT population should reflect the expected demographics of the target population(s) that are at greatest risk for systemic absorption—typically children, elderly, and those with greater disease severity.[48] The results of the MUsT may be used in different ways. For a topical formulation of an established systemic drug, the pharmokinetic (PK) results may be compared with those of the PK curve of the predetermined reference drug, to inform the understanding of relative risk of systemic adverse reactions and inform labeling decisions.[4] For drugs with a hormonal component, subjects are evaluated for HPA axis suppression, which may influence the benefit-risk assessment, particularly for younger patients. For NMEs, the MUsT may establish reference PK levels of systemic absorption for the drug. Examples of recently-approved dermatologic drugs whereby a MUsT was required as an element of the drug development program include minocycline 4% foam for acne (2019),[49] minocycline 1.5% foam for rosacea (2020),[50] tirbanibulin 1% ointment for actinic keratoses (2020),[51] and clascoterone 1% cream for acne (2020).[52] In the clascoterone MUsT, the increased incidence of HPA suppression in the subset of subjects aged 9 to 11 years was a contributing factor in limiting FDA approval of this drug to acne patients 12 years and older.[53]

New Drug Application/Biologic License Application Stage

Regulation

The *NDA/BLA stage* commences when a company submits to the FDA a comprehensive package[54] of the nonclinical and clinical studies conducted using the investigational drug for review and hopefully, approval for marketing. Before submission, the sponsor should request a *pre-NDA/BLA meeting*. The purpose of this meeting is to review the scope of the drug development program to ensure that there is sufficient evidence to enable DDD to make an informed assessment of the drug's efficacy and safety, and that there are no gaps in data. In addition, agreement should be reached on administrative details such as the order of contents, formats, or presentation of data. Preliminary discussions of risk management plans or postmarketing studies may also take place.[37]

Central to the submission of a marketing application is the requirement of demonstrating effectiveness, or "substantial evidence" that a product has an impact on the way a patient feels, functions, or survives. The 1997 FDA Modernization Act (FDAMA), codified in 21 USC 355, provides the statutory definition for "substantial evidence" of effectiveness that companies must demonstrate in order for a drug to be approved:

> ...evidence consisting of adequate and well-controlled investigations, including clinical investigations, by experts qualified by scientific training and experience to evaluate the effectiveness of the drug involved... that the drug will have the effect it purports ...to have under

---

[4]If the threshold level of systemic absorption for the reference drug that is necessary to cause an adverse reaction is unknown, those potential adverse reactions are included in the prescribing information for the topical drug, even if the PK levels are lower than the systemic drug.

Table 2 The FDA benefit-risk framework for human drug review[60]		
Dimension	**Evidence and Uncertainties**	**Conclusions and Reasons**
Analysis of Condition		
Current Treatment Options		
Benefit		
Risk and Risk Management		
Conclusions Regarding Benefit-Risk		

the conditions of use prescribed, recommended, or suggested in the labeling...[57]

Other requirements in the application necessary to assess the safety and reliability/product quality include a summary of safety information gained from clinical trials and a summary of chemistry, manufacturing, and controls (CMC). For biologics, immunogenicity studies are also included.

For a "standard" review, the DDD review team has 12 months from the date of submission to thoroughly review the NDA/BLA.[58] During the first 60 days, the team reviews the contents and quality of the sponsor's application for adequacy, consistent with the agreements made during the pre-NDA/BLA meeting. If the application is in order, it will be officially accepted ("filed") for review. Over the remaining 10 months, the members of the DDD team will individually perform analyses of the data to make their own determinations about the drug's efficacy and safety to ensure consistency with the sponsor's results, review quality control and manufacturing processes, conduct study and manufacturing site inspections, and identify any areas of uncertainty about any aspect of the drug. If questions arise during the DDD review, information requests (IRs) may be sent to the sponsor. The review team meets collectively at designated meetings during the review to share their findings with the group, discuss concerns, and build consensus about the overall benefit-risk assessment (BRA) and labeling of the drug at the proposed dose and indication.

The benefit-risk assessment framework[59] (**Table 2**) integrates the analysis of all the reviewers on the DDD team—clinical pharmacology, pharmacology and toxicology, CMC, biostatistics, and clinical—to provide a comprehensive evaluation of the evidence of clinical benefit to the target population, risks related to adverse reactions and product quality, and areas of uncertainty in the larger context of the seriousness or rarity of the disease and the extent of treatments available. If the BRA is favorable and approval recommended,

the team will then focus on the communication of this information to the patient and prescriber in the product labeling information.

Approval of the marketing application signifies that the FDA has determined that "the drug meets the statutory standards for safety and effectiveness, manufacturing and controls, and labeling."[61] If the review process reveals significant deficiencies in any of these areas, a Complete Response Letter (CRL) will be sent to the sponsor to explain why the statutory standards were not met, along with the elements required to resolve any deficiencies.[62] A CRL does not preclude future resubmission of the marketing application; however, the sponsor is strongly encouraged to request a meeting with the review team to clarify FDA expectations and discuss remediation.

Demonstrating substantial effectiveness in a rare disease

In 1983, Congress passed the Orphan Drug Act[63] to incentivize pharmaceutical companies to develop drugs for rare diseases, defined as one that affects less than 200,000 people in the US,[64] because most of these conditions do not have FDA-approved treatments. In addition, many of the 7000+ rare diseases are life-threatening and/or affect pediatric populations. For pharmaceutical companies, the small market size alone might discourage investment. There are also unique barriers to drug development for these small populations compared with more common dermatologic conditions, including greater uncertainty about the natural history and pathophysiology of the disease which can affect the development of appropriate inclusion criteria for subjects, trial design, and efficacy endpoints.[65] As noted earlier, the purpose of the FDA's Rare Disease Program is to raise the visibility and encourage the development of drugs for such conditions. Without specific treatments, clinicians often turn to off-label use of drugs that have not been tested in these patients, which may or may not have activity for the condition and may lead to unexpected adverse reactions.

Erythropoietic protoporphyria (EPP) is a rare genetic condition caused by a deficiency in ferrochelatase, the final enzyme in the heme synthesis pathway, leading to an accumulation of protoporphyrin IX (PPIX) in the skin, as well as in red blood cells and plasma. Clinically, this condition presents in childhood, when the affected patient experiences an immediate and severe phototoxic reaction when their skin is exposed to UVA sunlight (380–420 nm). Without treatment, the primary management strategy is sun avoidance, to include staying indoors in windowless rooms, sunprotective clothing, sunscreen, and over-the-counter antioxidants such as beta-carotene.

Afamelanotide, an α-melanocyte-stimulating hormone, which binds to the melanocortin-1 receptor (MC1R) which induces melanin synthesis and enhances DNA repair processes, was identified as a potential treatment of EPP. Clinically, the effect is to produce darkening of the skin, that is, stimulated photoprotection to better tolerate UV light. Because EPP is a rare disease, the sponsor requested and was granted several FDA statuses for afamelanotide to facilitate its development: orphan drug designation in 2008 and Fast Track designation in 2016. Early in the IND stage, the sponsor met several times with the FDA, including an EOP2 meeting in 2015, to discuss several issues unique to drugs being studied for rare diseases. Without the precedent of an approved treatment, novel endpoints need to be developed and validated for drugs. After the evaluation of the Phase 2 trial results, the sponsor and FDA agreed on an endpoint of "duration of direct sunlight exposure between [the hours of greatest intensity] on days when no pain was experienced" that was clinically meaningful,[66] but one that differed from the endpoint used in the Phase 2 trials.

A typical challenge for rare diseases is the small population of affected patients eligible to participate in clinical trials. For the afamelanotide Phase 3 trial, the sponsor could only enroll 94 EPP subjects. The FDA agreed that the results of this single Phase 3 pivotal trial, if favorable, along with supportive data from other clinical trials, would provide an adequate database for efficacy and safety. While the Phase 2 studies could not be considered "adequate and well-controlled" trials due to the post hoc change in the primary endpoint, the results could be supportive.[67] Ultimately, with the effect of afamelanotide increasing the duration of pain-free sun exposure in EPP subjects, the DDD consensus was that the evidence from the Phase 2 and 3 trials taken together was sufficient to demonstrate efficacy with an acceptable safety profile. Thus, afamelanotide was approved as a first-time treatment of EPP.

The benefit-risk assessment and communication and mitigation of risk

As previously mentioned, the decision of whether or not to recommend a dermatologic drug or biologic for approval rests on the integrated BRA of the DDD review team. Although the FDA framework provides a more structured and systematic approach to integrating the quantitative evidence, the BRA is largely qualitative,[68] and members of the review team may have different perspectives on the risks and benefits of a drug. It is not unusual for the review team to seek other perspectives within DDD or through consultation with other offices within CDER or other centers when there is overlapping jurisdiction. Occasionally, an issue during an IND or NDA/BLA review that could potentially affect or be impacted by FDA medical policy will be brought to the CDER Medical Policy and Program Council for senior management input, particularly if it involves class-level safety concerns or takes a position that might be precedent-setting, thus ensuring consistent implementation of policy.[69]

The Dermatologic and Ophthalmic Drugs Advisory Committee (DODAC), composed primarily of impartial medical specialists, typically physicians, is another source of expert opinion. In 2016, a unique safety concern of suicidal ideation and behavior (SIB) was identified during the drug development program of brodalumab, an interleukin-17 receptor A (IL-17A) blocker proposed for the treatment of moderate to severe psoriasis. While no causal association could be established between brodalumab and SIB, it was nonetheless troubling and the number of events occurring during development could not be dismissed. Considerable debate among the DDD review team occurred about how to weigh this adverse event into the benefit-risk assessment and the approval decision, especially in light of strong evidence of brodalumab's effectiveness and the recognized need to provide treatment alternatives for patients with moderate to severe psoriasis. It was noted that no psoriasis treatment is "universally effective for all patients and most severely affected patients generally lose response to the products they use over time."[70] To obtain additional perspectives and "independent expert advice that contributes to the quality of the agency's regulatory decision-making and lends credibility to the product review process,"[71] DDD brought these questions to the DODAC. The DODAC ultimately recommended approval of the biologic with the additional recommendations for prominent disclosure of these safety findings and a post-marketing risk management program. These recommendations from the DODAC, in addition to those from the Risk Evaluation and Mitigation Strategy (REMS) Oversight Committee, factored significantly into the decision to approve brodalumab as a second-line therapy for adult patients with moderate to severe plaque psoriasis who have failed other systemic therapies.[72]

For drugs such as brodalumab that demonstrate strong benefit but also pose an uncertain level of significant risk, gaining the support of an expert panel may not be enough to improve the benefit-risk balance. The primary means to tangibly improve the BRA is through risk mitigation. The prescribing information (PI, also known as labeling information) is the FDA's most visible method of communicating the benefits and risks of a drug. Communication of a serious risk can be strengthened through a black box warning. Although sufficient for most drugs, the PI is a passive means of risk mitigation. In addition, the label information may not be adequate to provide the context of the risk as it applies to an individual. Without this context, patients may not be able to make fully informed decisions about the drugs that are prescribed to them.[73]

In the case of brodalumab and SIB, FDA approval was contingent on the sponsor's implementation of a REMS, as recommended by the DODAC and the REMS Oversight Committee. The purpose of a risk management strategy is to mitigate an observed risk, thus ensuring that the benefits of a drug outweigh its risks.[74] A REM can also provide data to the sponsor, reportable to the FDA, about the real-world incidence of the adverse event being tracked. For the brodalumab REMS, prescriber/pharmacy education and certification, patient registry with documented patient counseling and consent, and a patient wallet card are some of the elements to assure safe use (ETASU)[75] of brodalumab.

Postmarketing Stage

After a marketing application for a drug has been approved, the sponsor has several immediate responsibilities. Before distributing the drug, the applicant must submit their final versions of the label, packaging, and promotional materials for approval. Any risk management programs required by the FDA (such as the REMS program for brodalumab due to the SIB risk) are implemented when the drug is marketed. In addition, any postmarketing requirements (PMRs) required (such as deferred pediatric studies) or postmarketing commitments (PMCs) agreed on during the

NDA/BLA review should be initiated. Finally, for NMEs and biologics, the applicant may request a postapproval feedback meeting with the FDA. This meeting is an opportunity to discuss the quality of the application, evaluate the communication process during drug development and marketing application review, and learn from what was successful and whereby improvement could be made in future drug programs.

Besides these immediate obligations, the applicant must continue long-term safety surveillance of the drug in accordance with 21 CFR 314.80, and submit quarterly reports of adverse events.[76] While the number of subjects enrolled in the Phase 3 trials may have been enough to detect the most common adverse reactions of a drug, long-term surveillance is necessary to monitor for less common adverse reactions. Rare adverse events may not be observed until the drug has been prescribed to a larger population or has been taken for longer periods of time. Adverse events that are serious and unexpected must be reported to the FDA in a timely manner, that is, in a 7- or 15-day safety report.

The applicant must also submit a comprehensive annual report of the drug development program to the FDA, including a status of the PMRs/PMCs, adverse events, additional nonclinical studies conducted, anticipated shortages, and future plans to study or modify aspects of the drug (e.g., manufacturing process).[77] The applicant may continue to study its efficacy in other indications and in other populations. In some cases, the nonclinical studies previously conducted during the pre-IND stage will still be applicable to these new clinical studies, shortening the developmental pathway to approval. Assuming that the drug formulation and strength/concentration do not change, the company may continue to submit additional IND studies for any phase of clinical study (1, 2, or 3), depending on what other supporting clinical studies have been completed in and outside of the United States. Applications for approval for expanded indications or for additional populations are submitted as supplemental NDAs (sNDAs) or supplemental BLAs (sBLAs).

SPECIAL TOPICS OF DERMATOLOGIC CONCERN
Protecting Children Through Research

Although 21 CFR 50 Subpart D allows for clinical investigations in children,[78] until the late 1990s clinical testing in pediatric subjects was infrequently conducted for several reasons: ethical concerns about subjecting this vulnerable population to unknown safety risks, inability for the subjects to give informed consent, extra care necessary to ensure children can be compliant with study procedures, and the perceived lack of necessity. The consensus in the medical community was to protect children by minimizing exposure to drugs under development. Thus, only about 20% of drugs under development were studied in children.[79] However, with so few drugs approved and available for pediatric use, physicians in clinical practice had no option but to treat children like "small adults" by extrapolating in a trial-and-error fashion from adult indications and dosages.[79] Anecdotal reports of adverse reactions occurring from off-label use of drugs in children increased the visibility of this issue.

Currently, the FDA has two means to maximize clinical testing of drugs under development intended for pediatric patients. Under the 1997 Best Pharmaceuticals for Children Act (BPCA), the FDA provides an incentive of up to 6 months of additional marketing exclusivity for a drug if the sponsor voluntarily conducts studies in children. In contrast, the Pediatric Research Equity Act (PREA),[80] gives the FDA the authority to require that pediatric studies be conducted if a sponsor is seeking FDA approval with a new active ingredient, indication, dosage form, dosing regimen, or route of administration, unless a waiver or deferral has been approved. This requirement ensures that whereby appropriate and practicable, drugs are developed in appropriate formulations for children, and that accurate pediatric safety and dosing information is included in labeling.[81] During development, discussion of pediatric study plans takes place no later than the EOP2 meeting. Within 60 days after the EOP2 meeting, the sponsor must submit an initial pediatric study plan (iPSP), or at least 120 days before a Phase 3 protocol submission if there was no EOP2 meeting.[82] For systemic drugs, a sponsor may request a deferral until the postmarketing stage to first characterize a drug's safety profile in adults, or a waiver for certain age groups if there are safety concerns or if studies are highly impracticable.[81]

Compared with older systemic drugs such as methotrexate and cyclosporine that have long been prescribed to treat severe dermatologic diseases such as psoriasis and atopic dermatitis, biologics have revolutionized treatment by offering rapid improvement with relatively few adverse reactions by selectively targeting aberrant proteins in specific inflammatory pathways. One of the first biologics to treat plaque psoriasis, etanercept, was first approved for adults in 2004. Although it was the first biologic approved for adolescents with psoriasis, that approval took more than 12 years due to early uncertainties related to potential drug-induced malignancy in children with long-term use. Similar safety concerns also sidetracked the study of adalimumab for pediatric psoriasis. Nonetheless, due to the significant unmet need for effective systemic therapies to treat severe skin disease in children and an ethical evolution that "the best way to bolster outcomes and protect children is through research, not from research,"[83] DDD now encourages the conduct of pediatric clinical studies earlier during the development of drugs that treat chronic dermatologic conditions affecting children. This change is most evident with the approval dates of the biologics, with a significant reduction in the time interval between approval dates for adults and those for children (**Table 3**). DDD has also authored several guidances for specific pediatric diseases to improve the transparency about FDA

Table 3
Time interval between adult and pediatric approvals for biologics used in dermatology[84]

Biologic	Indication	FDA approval Date for Adults	FDA Approval Date(s) for Pediatrics[a]	Time Interval Between Adult and Pediatric Approval(s)
Etanercept	Plaque psoriasis	Apr 2004	Nov 2016: 4–17 y	12 years, 7 months
Adalimumab	Plaque psoriasis	Jan 2008	Not FDA-approved	N/A
Ustekinumab	Plaque psoriasis	Sep 2009	Oct 2017: 12 to <17 y	6 years, 1 month
			Jul 2020: 6 to <12 y	8 years, 9 month
Adalimumab	Hidradenitis suppurativa	Sep 2015	Oct 2018: 12 to <17 y	3 years, 1 month
Ixekizumab	Plaque psoriasis	Mar 2016	Mar 2020: 6 to <17 y	4 years
Dupilumab	Atopic dermatitis	Mar 2017	Mar 2019: 12 to<17 y	2 years
			May 2020: 6 to <12 y	3 years, 2 months

[a] These dates refer only to the specified indication.

expectations about pediatric clinical trials and encourage sponsors to develop drugs for these indications (see Appendix 2).

Biosimilars

Due to the complexity of their structures and multiple indications which necessitate multiple patents, biologics enjoy a patent exclusivity period of at least 12 years, which can be extended through approval for additional indications and other minor modifications. With the expiration of the core US patents for etanercept, adalimumab, and ustekinumab approaching, biosimilars have become a rapidly expanding category of medical products coming under review in DDD. Although biosimilars have a phased development program and marketing application process described in 42 U.S C. 262 that is loosely analogous to the one for drugs and biologics, the statutory requirement for biosimilar approval is "demonstration of biosimilarity"[85] to a reference product (the branded biologic). Unlike drugs and biologics whereby the sponsor must conduct separate clinical efficacy and safety trials as evidence of effectiveness for each indication, the FDA recommends a stepwise, scientifically grounded approach to establish biosimilarity in a single indication (eg, psoriasis) through:

- Analytical comparability
- Animal studies (including toxicity)
- PK, pharmacodynamic, and immunogenicity assessments against a reference product
- Comparative clinical study with a reference product as the comparator in a single indication (e.g., psoriasis)[86]

If the FDA agrees that the sponsor has successfully demonstrated that the biosimilar is "highly similar" with "no clinically meaningful differences...in terms of safety, purity, and potency,"[85] then the sponsor may seek extrapolation to all other FDA-approved indications for the reference product, including pediatric indications, without conducting additional studies. Sponsors may not seek approval for indications that are still under exclusivity protection or make modifications to their product that go beyond what has already been established by the reference product.

SUMMARY

By virtue of its regulatory authority invested by the FD&CA, the FDA is the ultimate arbiter of drug approval in the United States, and for dermatologic drugs specifically, the Division of Dermatology and Dentistry in CDER. As a science-led organization, FDA uses the best scientific and technological information available to make benefit-risk decisions through a deliberative process. At the same time, by engaging with other stakeholders in drug development, DDD is a partner in expanding the therapeutic options for the diverse patient population affected by dermatologic conditions. We welcome frequent and open dialogue with sponsors about their drug development programs to provide timely feedback and guidance, while staying attuned to what is considered clinically meaningful to the patients who will ultimately take the drug. By constantly reassessing the parameters of risk and benefit in the context of dermatologic disease, DDD is committed to maintain the public trust in the safety and efficacy of FDA-approved drugs.

ACKNOWLEDGMENTS

The authors acknowledge the assistance of Julie Bietz, MD; Hon Sum Ko, MD; Barbara Hill, PhD; and Chinmay Shukla, PhD. The authors received no financial support for the research, authorship, and/or publication of this article.

DECLARATION OF CONFLICTING INTERESTS

The authors declared no potential conflicts of interest with respect to research, authorship, and/or publication of this article.

SUPPLEMENTARY DATA

Supplementary data related to this article can be found online at https://doi.org/10.1016/j.det.2022.02.001.

REFERENCES

1. Food and Drug Administration. What We Do. Available at: https://www.fda.gov/about-fda/what-we-do. Accessed January 21, 2021.
2. Institute of Medicine (US). Forum on drug discovery, development, and Translation. Challenges for the FDA: the future of drug safety, workshop summary. Washington, DC: The National Academies Press; 2007. Available at: https://www.ncbi.nlm.nih.gov/books/NBK52919/. Accessed March 15, 2021.
3. Taylor D. The pharmaceutical industry and the future of drug development. In: Hester RE, Harrison RM, editors. Pharmaceuticals in the environment. The Royal Society of Chemistry; 2016. p. 1–33. Available at: https://pubs.rsc.org/en/content/chapterhtml/2015/bk9781782621898-00001?isbn=978-1-78262-189-8. Accessed March 29, 2021.
4. Wong CH, Siah KW, Lo AW. Estimation of clinical trial success rates and related parameters. Biostatistics

2019;20(2):273–86 [published correction appears in Biostatistics. ;20(2):366].

5. Olsen AK, Whalen MD. Public perceptions of the pharmaceutical industry and drug safety: implications for the pharmacovigilance professional and the culture of safety. Drug Saf 2009;32(10): 805–10.

6. Mohs RC, Greig NH. Drug discovery and development: Role of basic biological research. Alzheimers Dement (N Y) 2017;3(4):651–7.

7. Koay PP, Sharp RR. The role of patient advocacy organizations in shaping genomic science. Annu Rev Genomics Hum Genet 2013;14:579–95.

8. Altman DJ. The roles of the pharmaceutical industry and drug development in dermatology and dermatologic health care. Dermatol Clin 2000;18(2): 287–96.

9. Davari M, Khorasani E, Tigabu BM. Factors influencing prescribing decisions of physicians: A review. Ethiop J Health Sci 2018;28(6):795–804.

10. Latten T, Westra D, Angeli F, et al. Pharmaceutical companies and healthcare providers: Going beyond the gift - An explorative review. PLoS One 2018; 13(2):e0191856.

11. Lowe MM, Blaser DA, Cone L, et al. Increasing patient involvement in drug development. Value Health 2016;19(6):869–78.

12. Health Literacy. National Institutes of Health. Available at: https://www.nih.gov/institutes-nih/nih-office-director/office-communications-public-liaison/clear-communication/health-literacy. Accessed 29 March 2021.

13. Koh HK, Brach C, Harris LM, et al. A proposed 'health literate care model' would constitute a systems approach to improving patients' engagement in care. Health Aff (Millwood) 2013;32(2):357–67.

14. Aikin KJ, Swasy JL, Braman AC. Patient and Physician Attitudes and Behaviors Associated With DTC Promotion of Prescription Drugs —Summary of FDA Survey Research Results, Final Report. Center for Drug Evaluation and Research, Food and Drug Administration, US Dept of Health and Human Services; 2004.

15. Stein S, Bogard E, Boice N, et al. Principles for interactions with biopharmaceutical companies: the development of guidelines for patient advocacy organizations in the field of rare diseases. Orphanet J Rare Dis 2018;13(1):18.

16. Rose SL, Highland J, Karafa MT, et al. Patient advocacy organizations, industry funding, and conflicts of interest. JAMA Intern Med 2017;177(3):344–50.

17. Fabbri A, Parker L, Colombo C, et al. Industry funding of patient and health consumer organisations: systematic review with meta-analysis. BMJ 2020; 368:l6925.

18. Collins S. The growing importance of incorporating US payers into biotechnology drug development decision-making. J Commer Biotechnol 2011;17: 151–8. https://doi.org/10.1057/jcb.2010.29.

19. Bergthold LA. Medical necessity: do we need it? Health Aff (Millwood) 1995;14(4):180–90.

20. See 42 U.S.C. 1395y. Available at: https://uscode.house.gov/view.xhtml?req=(title:42%20section:1395y%20edition:prelim.

21. Doux J. Barriers and opportunities: A view across the developmental divide. J Invest Dermatol 2015; 135(9):2143–4.

22. Food and Drug Administration. Rare Diseases Program. Available at: https://www.fda.gov/about-fda/center-drug-evaluation-and-research-cder/rare-diseases-program. Accessed February 13, 2021.

23. Food and Drug Administration. CDER Patient-Focused Drug Development. Available at: https://www.fda.gov/drugs/development-approval-process-drugs/cder-patient-focused-drug-development. Accessed February 13, 2021.

24. The Voice of the Patient: Alopecia Areata. Center for Drug Evaluation and Research, Food and Drug Administration, US Dept of Health and Human Services. 2018. Available at: https://www.fda.gov/media/112100/download. Accessed February 13, 2021.

25. Gorlin Syndrome Alliance. Report of FDA Gorlin Syndrome Patient-Led Listening Session 11/09/2020. Available at: https://gorlinsyndrome.org/report-of-fda-gorlin-syndrome-patient-led-listening-session-11-09-2020/. Accessed February 13, 2021.

26. Drug Amendments of 1962, Federal Food, Drug, and Cosmetic Act;1962:780-796. Available at: https://www.govinfo.gov/content/pkg/STATUTE-76/pdf/STATUTE-76-Pg780.pdf. Accessed January 21, 2021.

27. Food and Drug Administration. What We Do. Available at: https://www.fda.gov/about-fda/what-we-do. Accessed January 21, 2021.

28. See 21 U.S.C. 355. Available at: https://uscode.house.gov/view.xhtml?hl=false&edition=prelim&req=granuleid%3AUSC-prelim-title21-section355&num=0&saved=%7CZ3JhbnVsZWlkOIVTQy1wcmVsaW0tdGl0bGUyMS1zZWN0aW9uMzU1%7C%7C%7C0%7Cfalse%7Cprelim.

29. See 21 CFR 312 and 21 CFR 314. Available at: https://www.ecfr.gov/cgi-bin/text-idx?SID=7dc63ae09b575d718ea123da1bc9a729&mc=true&tpl=/ecfrbrowse/Title21/21cfrv5_02.tpl#0.

30. See the guidance for industry Best Practices for Communication Between IND Sponsors and FDA During Drug Development (December 2017). We update guidances periodically. For the most recent version of a guidance. check the FDA guidance web page at Available at: https://www.fda.gov/regulatory-information/search-fda-guidance-documents.

31. See the guidance for industry Best Practices for Communication Between IND Sponsors and FDA During Drug Development. 2017. Available at.

https://www.fda.gov/regulatory-information/search-fda-guidance-documents.

32. See 21 CFR 312.21. Available at: https://www.ecfr.gov/cgi-bin/text-idx?SID=c3bdad24b0db85d1fe6585019c370e6e&mc=true&node=sp21.5.312.b&rgn=div6.

33. A search engine is available on the FDA guidance web page at. https://www.fda.gov/regulatory-information/search-fda-guidance-documents.

34. See 21 CFR 312.47. Available at: https://www.ecfr.gov/cgi-bin/text-idx?SID=f644fb5c6edb39d975f3c1bff6febc44&mc=true&node=se21.5.312_147&rgn=div8.

35. See the guidance for industry M3(R2) Nonclinical Safety Studies for the Conduct of Human Clinical Trials and Marketing Authorization for Pharmaceuticals (January 2010). Available at: https://www.fda.gov/regulatory-information/search-fda-guidance-documents.

36. See guidance for industry IND Meetings for Human Drugs and Biologics: Chemistry, Manufacturing, and Controls Information. 2001. Available at. https://www.fda.gov/regulatory-information/search-fda-guidance-documents.

37. See FDA's MAPP 6030.9 Good Review Practice: Good Review Management Principles and Practices for Effective IND Development and Review (April 2019).

38. Chandra SA, Stokes AH, Hailey R, et al. Dermal toxicity studies: factors impacting study interpretation and outcome. Toxicol Pathol 2015;43(4):474–81.

39. Sandberg B. Topical Drug Products: US FDA, Experts tackle challenges of dermal safety studies. Web site. 2018. Available at: https://pink.pharmaintelligence.informa.com/PS123855/Topical-Drug-Products-US-FDA-Experts-Tackle-Challenges-Of-Dermal-Safety-Studies. Accessed March 2, 2021.

40. See draft guidance for industry Contact Dermatitis from Topical Drug Products for Cutaneous Application: Human Safety Assessment (March 2020). When final, this guidance will represent the FDA's current thinking on this topic.

41. Avila AM, Bebenek I, Bonzo JA, et al. An FDA/CDER perspective on nonclinical testing strategies: Classical toxicology approaches and new approach methodologies (NAMs). Regul Toxicol Pharmacol 2020;114:104662.

42. Food and Drug Administration. FDA's Predictive Toxicology Roadmap. Available at: https://www.fda.gov/media/109634/download. Accessed February 12, 2021.

43. Food and Drug Administration. Advancing Alternative Methods at FDA. Available at: https://www.fda.gov/science-research/about-science-research-fda/advancing-alternative-methods-fda. Accessed February 12, 2021.

44. See guidance for industry FDA Acceptance of Foreign Clinical Studies Not Conducted Under an IND Frequently Asked Questions. 2012. Available at: https://www.fda.gov/regulatory-information/search-fda-guidance-documents.

45. Lu H, Rosenbaum S. Developmental pharmacokinetics in pediatric populations. J Pediatr Pharmacol Ther 2014;19(4):262–76.

46. Klotz U. Pharmacokinetics and drug metabolism in the elderly. Drug Metab Rev 2009;41(2):67–76.

47. Dhar S, Seth J, Parikh D. Systemic side-effects of topical corticosteroids. Indian J Dermatol 2014;59(5):460–4.

48. Bashaw ED, Tran DC, Shukla CG, et al. Maximal usage trial: An overview of the design of systemic bioavailability trial for topical dermatological products. Ther Innov Regul Sci 2015;49(1):108–15.

49. See FDA Multi-discipline review for Amzeeq (minocycline topical foam 4%) (NDA 212379), dated October 18, 2019, available on the Drugs @FDA web page at. Available at: https://www.accessdata.fda.gov/scripts/cder/daf/index.cfm.

50. See FDA Multi-discipline review for Zilxi (minocycline topical foam, 1.5%)(NDA 213690), dated May 22, 2020, available on the Drugs @FDA web page at. Available at: https://www.accessdata.fda.gov/scripts/cder/daf/index.cfm.

51. See FDA Multi-discipline review for Klisyri (tirbanibulin ointment 1%)(NDA 213189), dated December 9, 2020, available on the Drugs @FDA web page at. Available at: https://www.accessdata.fda.gov/scripts/cder/daf/index.cfm.

52. See FDA Multi-discipline review for Winlevi (clascoterone cream 1%)(NDA213433) dated August 26, 2020, available on the Drugs @FDA web page at. Available at: https://www.accessdata.fda.gov/scripts/cder/daf/index.cfm.

53. See Sec 6.2.1.2, FDA Multi-discipline review for Winlevi (clascoterone cream 1%)(NDA213433) dated August 26, 2020, available on the Drugs @FDA web page at. Available at: https://www.accessdata.fda.gov/scripts/cder/daf/index.cfm.

54. See 21 CFR 314.50. Available at: https://www.ecfr.gov/cgi-bin/text-idx?SID=674dc6cad29846d3d06f4426a72d2436&mc=true&node=pt21.5.314&rgn=div5#se21.5.314_150.

57. See 21 U.S.C. 355(d). Available at: https://uscode.house.gov/view.xhtml?req=granuleid:USC-prelim-title21-section355&num=0&edition=prelim.

58. Food and Drug Administration. CDER 21st Century Review Process Desk Reference Guide. Available at. https://www.fda.gov/media/78941/download.

59. The key considerations and common sources of uncertainty in the BRA are described in great detail in Benefit-Risk Assessment Throughout the Drug Lifecycle: FDA Discussion Document. 2019. Available at. https://healthpolicy.duke.edu/sites/default/

files/2020-07/discussion_guide_b-r_assessment_may16_0.pdf.

60. The Duke-Margolis Center for Health Policy. Advancing Structured Benefit-Risk Assessment in FDA Review. Washington, DC. 2017. Available at. https://healthpolicy.duke.edu/sites/default/files/2020-03/structured_b-r_discussion_guide%20%281%29.pdf.

61. See 21 CFR 314.105. Available at: https://www.accessdata.fda.gov/scripts/cdrh/cfdocs/cfcfr/CFRSearch.cfm?fr=314.105.

62. See 21 CFR 314.110. Available at: https://www.accessdata.fda.gov/scripts/cdrh/cfdocs/cfcfr/cfrsearch.cfm?fr=314.110#:~:text=A%20complete%20response%20letter%20reflects,that%20the%20agency%20has%20reviewed.

63. See 21 CFR 316 Available at. https://www.ecfr.gov/cgi-bin/text-idx?c=ecfr&SID=51cf70689d51f0ea4147c0a8ac649321&rgn=div5&view=text&node=21:5.0.1.1.6&idno=21#sp21.5.316.

64. Food and Drug Administration. Orphan Drug Act – Relevant Excerpts. Available at: https://www.fda.gov/industry/designating-orphan-product-drugs-and-biological-products/orphan-drug-act-relevant-excerpts. Accessed February 13, 2021.

65. See draft guidance for industry Rare Diseases: Natural History Studies for Drug Development (March 2019). When final, this guidance will represent the FDA's current thinking on this topic.

66. Scientific Workshop on Erythropoietic Protoporphyria (EPP) Summary Report. Food and Drug Administration, US Dept of Health and Human Services; 2017.

67. See FDA Multi-Discipline Review for Scenesse (afamelanotide)(NDA 210797), dated October 8, 2019, available on the Drugs @FDA web page at. Available at: https://www.accessdata.fda.gov/scripts/cder/daf/index.cfm.

68. Angelis A, Phillips LD. Advancing structured decision-making in drug regulation at the FDA and EMA. Br J Clin Pharmacol 2021;87(2):395–405.

69. See FDA's MAPP 4301.1 Rev 3, Center for Drug Evaluation and Research Medical Policy Council, February 2021.

70. See FDA Summary Review for Siliq (brodalumab) (BLA 761032) dated February 6, 2017, available on the Drugs @FDA web page at. https://www.accessdata.fda.gov/scripts/cder/daf/index.cfm.

71. Food and Drug Administration. Advisory Committees: Critical to the FDA's Product Review Process. Available at: https://www.fda.gov/drugs/information-consumers-and-patients-drugs/advisory-committees-critical-fdas-product-review-process. Accessed February 13, 2021.

72. See FDA Summary Review for Siliq (brodalumab) (BLA 761032) dated February 6, 2017, available on the Drugs @FDA web page at. Available at: https://www.accessdata.fda.gov/scripts/cder/daf/index.cfm.

73. Food and Drug Administration. Strategic Plan for Risk Communication. Available at: https://www.fda.gov/about-fda/reports/strategic-plan-risk-communication. Accessed April 12, 2021.

74. See guidance for industry REMS. FDA's Application of Statutory Factors in Determining When a REMS is Necessary (April 2019). Available at. https://www.fda.gov/regulatory-information/search-fda-guidance-documents.

75. FDA Risk Evaluation and Mitigation Strategy (REMS) Document - SILIQ® (brodalumab) REMS Program. Available at. https://www.accessdata.fda.gov/drugsatfda_docs/rems/Siliq_2021_01_22_REMS_Full.pdf. Accessed April 12, 2021.

76. See 21 CFR 314.80. Available at. https://www.accessdata.fda.gov/scripts/cdrh/cfdocs/cfcfr/CFRSearch.cfm?fr=314.80.

77. See 21 CFR 314.81. Available at: https://www.accessdata.fda.gov/scripts/cdrh/cfdocs/cfcfr/CFRSearch.cfm?fr=314.81.

78. See 21 CFR 50. Available at: https://www.ecfr.gov/cgi-bin/text-idx?SID=e95ffa4de60df1f03420179179dcc049&mc=true&node=sp21.1.50.d&rgn=div6.

79. Food and Drug Administration. Drug Research and Children. Available at: https://www.fda.gov/drugs/information-consumers-and-patients-drugs/drug-research-and-children. Accessed April 5, 2021.

80. See 21 U.S.C. 355c. Available at: https://uscode.house.gov/view.xhtml?req=granuleid:USC-prelim-title21-section355c&num=0&edition=prelim.

81. See draft guidance for industry How to Comply with the Pediatric Research Equity Act (September 2005). When final, this guidance will represent the FDA's current thinking on this topic.

82. See guidance for industry Pediatric Study Plans: Content of and Process for Submitting Initial Pediatric Study Plans and Amended Initial Pediatric Study Plans. 2020. Available at: https://www.fda.gov/regulatory-information/search-fda-guidance-documents.

83. Lowenthal E, Fiks AG. Protecting children through research. Editorial Pediatr 2016;138(4):e20162150.

84. These timelines were compiled from the approval dates of these drugs, available at Drugs@FDA: FDA-Approved Drugs. Available at: https://www.accessdata.fda.gov/scripts/cder/daf/index.cfm?event=overview.process&ApplNo=103795.

85. See 42 U.S.C. 262. Available at: https://uscode.house.gov/view.xhtml?req=granuleid:USC-prelim-title42-section262&num=0&edition=prelim.

86. See guidance to industry Scientific Considerations in Demonstrating Biosimiliarity to a Reference Product. April 2015). Available at: https://www.fda.gov/regulatory-information/search-fda-guidance-documents.

Postmarket Assessment for Drugs and Biologics Used in Dermatology and Cutaneous Adverse Drug Reactions

Melissa Reyes, MD, MPH[a,b,*], Cindy Kortepeter, PharmD[a],
Monica Muñoz, PharmD, PhD, BCPS[a]

KEYWORDS

- Postmarket surveillance • Cutaneous adverse drug reactions • Severe cutaneous adverse reactions
- Stevens–Johnson syndrome • Toxic epidermal necrolysis • Adverse event reporting

KEY POINTS

- The US Food and Drug Administration maintains a system of postmarketing surveillance programs to identify and evaluate new safety concerns after a drug's approval.
- Dermatologists play a critical role in identifying, managing, and reporting adverse events associated with dermatologic treatments and cutaneous adverse events.
- Postmarketing adverse event reports have been particularly vital in the detection and evaluation of serious cutaneous adverse reactions and resulting risk mitigation actions, such as labeling changes.

INTRODUCTION

The US Food and Drug Administration (FDA) Center for Drug Evaluation and Research (CDER) ensures that safe and effective drugs are available to improve the health of individuals in the United States.[1] To fulfill this mission, the CDER balances the promotion of drug development, the availability of high-quality drugs for patients, and the maintenance of a favorable benefit/risk profile for approved drugs[2] through risk management, a combination of risk assessment and risk minimization.[3] Pharmacovigilance, "the science and activities relating to the detection, assessment, understanding and prevention of adverse effects or any other drug related problems,"[4] informs the CDER's risk management of drugs using a variety of postmarketing safety data sources to identify new safety signals and conduct risk assessments

to continually assess the benefit-to-risk profile of a regulated drug.[4]

Cutaneous adverse drug reactions (CADR) are reported to be one of the most frequently reported adverse events occurring in patients undergoing drug therapy, ranging between 1% and 3% in hospitalized patients and from 10 to 38% of all reported adverse drug reactions (ADR).[5,6] Morbilliform eruptions account for approximately 95% of all CADR.[7] Stevens-Johnson syndrome (SJS) and toxic epidermal necrolysis (TEN) are the concerning CADRs, with significant morbidity and mortality. In the general population, events of SJS/TEN are uncommon, estimated between 1 and 2 cases per million people for TEN and between 1 and 7 cases per million people for SJS, although SJS may occur at higher rates in the United States (≤ 9.2 cases per million people).[8] Uncommon adverse events such as SJS/TEN are

[a] Division of Pharmacovigilance, Food and Drug Administration, Center for Drug Evaluation and Research, Office of Surveillance and Epidemiology, 10903 New Hampshire Avenue, Silver Spring, MD 20993, USA;
[b] Department of Dermatology, Uniformed Services University of the Health Sciences
* Corresponding author. 10903 New Hampshire Avenue, Silver Spring, MD 20993.
E-mail address: Melissa.Reyes@fda.hhs.gov

Dermatol Clin 40 (2022) 265–277
https://doi.org/10.1016/j.det.2022.02.002
0733-8635/22/Published by Elsevier Inc.

unlikely to occur during the preapproval studies given the size of the study population; thus, the potential risk of for SJS/TEN is usually unknown at the time of drug approval. The identification of an uncommon adverse event may occur once the drug is broadly used in a larger population.[9]

The identification of new safety issues using spontaneous adverse event reporting is based on the clinical observations made at the patient–health care provider level.[10] In dermatology, spontaneous adverse event reports have resulted in regulatory actions for drugs prescribed by dermatologists for cutaneous disorders, such as efalizumab for psoriasis,[11] and CADR, such as chemical leukoderma with the use of the methylphenidate transdermal system.[12]

The involvement of dermatologists in pharmacovigilance is of increasing importance as the number of drugs being investigated for dermatologic conditions is increasing[13] and a variety of life-threatening and non–life-threatening CADRs have been reported.[14–16] In the American Academy of Dermatology's 1996 Guidelines of Care for Cutaneous Adverse Reactions, under the heading *Recommendations–Miscellaneous,* the authors' advise that adverse drug reactions "may be voluntarily reported to the manufacturer or to" the FDA.[17] Dermatologists, as the prescriber of several newly approved drugs or in consultation with patients with suspected serious, uncommon CADR such as SJS/TEN, play a valuable and critical role in identifying important, new drug safety information in the postmarketing period.

The goal of this article is to describe the FDA's postmarket surveillance of drugs and highlight the important role of dermatologists in pharmacovigilance.

DEFINITIONS

Approval: For ease of reference, this article uses the term approval to refer to both drug approval and biologic licensure.

Applicant: The company that submits an application to the FDA for approval to market a drug product in the United States.[18]

Drug: For ease of reference, this article uses the term drug to refer to all human drug and therapeutic biological products regulated by the CDER.

Label: Any display of written, printed, or graphic matter on the immediate container of any article, or any such matter affixed to any consumer commodity or affixed to or appearing on a package containing any consumer commodity.[19]

Labeling: Includes all written, printed, or graphic matter accompanying an article at any time while such article is in interstate commerce or held for sale after shipment or delivery in interstate commerce.[19]

Pharmacovigilance: "The science and activities relating to the detection, assessment, understanding and prevention of adverse effects or any other possible drug-related problems."[20]

Risk evaluation and mitigation strategy: "A Risk Evaluation and Mitigation Strategy, or REMS, is a safety plan to manage a known or potential serious risk associated with a medicine and to enable patients to have continued access to such medicines by managing their safe use."[18]

Safety signal: Information from 1 or more sources that suggests a new potential causal association, or a new aspect of a known association, between a drug and an adverse event that warrants further action to verify.[21,22]

Serious adverse drug experience: "Any adverse drug experience occurring at any dose that results in any of the following outcomes: Death, a life-threatening adverse drug experience, inpatient hospitalization or prolongation of existing hospitalization, a persistent or significant disability/incapacity, or a congenital anomaly/birth defect. Important medical events that may not result in death, be life-threatening, or require hospitalization may be considered a serious adverse drug experience when, based upon appropriate medical judgment, they may jeopardize the patient or subject and may require medical or surgical intervention to prevent one of the outcomes listed in this definition."[23]

DISCUSSION
US Food and Drug Administration Postmarketing Surveillance of Drugs

Pharmacovigilance began in the mid-19th century and has evolved into a global effort as the manufacture and distribution of drugs has changed. A brief timeline highlighting the history of drug safety regulation in the United States is provided in **Table 1**.[24-26]

The US Code of Federal Regulations defines the Applicant's responsibilities to conduct postmarketing surveillance for medical products (21 CFR §314.80 and §600.80 for approved drugs and biological products, respectively), and the Food, Drug & Cosmetics Act outlines the FDA's duty[27]; postmarketing surveillance is a shared responsibility, and the focus of this discussion is on the FDA's surveillance practices.

The CDER regulates drugs, which includes over-the-counter and prescription drugs, as well as biological therapeutics and generic drugs. Drugs, as defined by regulation, also includes antiperspirants, dandruff shampoos, and sunscreen.[28]

Table 1
Milestones in the US FDA's regulation of drug safety

1938	The Federal Food, Drug, and Cosmetic (FDC) Act creates a new public health system requiring new drugs to be shown safe prior to marketing.
1951	The Durham–Humphrey Amendment defines drugs that cannot be used safely without medical supervision and restricts the sale of these drugs by requiring prescription by a licensed practitioner.
1966	The Fair Packaging and Labeling Act requires consumer products to be honestly and informatively labeled, with the FDA enforcing requirements on drugs among other products.
1970	In Upjohn v Finch, the Court of Appeals rules that commercial success alone does not constitute substantial evidence of drug safety and efficacy, upholding the enforcement of the 1962 Kefauver–Harris Drug Amendments.
1993	The FDA introduces MedWatch to facilitate the voluntary reporting by health care professionals to the FDA of adverse events that may be due to FDA regulated drugs and devices.
1998	The Adverse Event Reporting System (AERS), a computerized information database to support postmarketing surveillance is introduced.
2005	The FDA publishes 3 guidances describing the processes for the risk management of regulated drugs.
2006	The FDA approves the final rule "Requirements on Content and Format of Labeling for Human Prescription Drug and Biological Products" to improve the usability of FDA-approved labeling by health care professionals.
2007	Title IX, section 915 of The FDA Amendments Act (FDAAA) grants the FDA the authority to require Applicants to conduct postmarketing studies to enhance understanding of drug safety, require Applicants to comply with Risk Evaluation and Mitigation Strategies (REMS), and enforce safety-related label changes. FDAAA also requires the FDA to prepare summary analysis of adverse drug reaction reports received by 18 mo post-approval or after use of the drug by 10,000 individuals, whichever is later of any new risks not previously identified, potential new risks, or unknown risks reported in unusual number. In addition, FDAAA requires regular, biweekly screening of AERS and quarterly posting of any new safety information or potential signal of a serious risk identified by AERS within the last quarter.
2016	21st Century Cures Act (Cures Act) eliminates the requirement for the FDA summary analyses for drugs and adds a requirement for the FDA to make publicly available guidelines describing best practice for drug safety surveillance using the FAERS and criteria for public posting of adverse event signals. In addition, the Cures Act removes the requirement for biweekly screening and summary analysis of the FAERS as required by FDAAA.

Within the CDER, the Office of Surveillance and Epidemiology monitors and evaluates the safety of drugs using a variety of safety experts and surveillance tools throughout the life cycle of the drugs[29] along with the divisions that regulate premarket, drug development programs and drug approvals. The Office of Surveillance and Epidemiology includes the Divisions of Pharmacovigilance, the Divisions of Epidemiology, and the Office of Medication Error Prevention and Risk Management. The Divisions of Pharmacovigilance's safety teams are composed of medical officers and safety evaluators with each team assigned a portfolio of therapeutic drug classes, collectively covering all approved drugs.[30] The procedures for how the Office of Surveillance and Epidemiology conducts postmarketing surveillance are outlined in a variety of internal and external documents[3,4,26] and describes the processes for the monitoring of *adverse events*, defined as:

any untoward medical occurrence associated with the use of a drug product in humans, whether or not it is considered related to the drug product. An adverse event can occur in the course of the use of a drug product; from overdose of a drug product, whether accidental or intentional; from abuse of a drug product; from discontinuation of the drug product (eg, physiologic withdrawal); and it includes any failure of expected pharmacologic action.[31]

Data Sources for Postmarketing Surveillance

During postmarketing surveillance, safety signals can arise from various data sources. The source of a signal typically includes spontaneous reports to the FDA and medical literature but can also come from a variety of other sources, including postmarket studies.[21,22,26] Upon identification of a safety signal, a comprehensive, in-depth assessment of the drug–adverse event combination is initiated.

US Food and Drug Administration Adverse Event Reporting System

The FDA's Adverse Event Reporting System (FAERS) contains information on adverse event and medication error reports submitted to the FDA in the format of individual case safety reports. Since its inception in 1968, as of December 31, 2021, the FAERS contained 23,663,780 total reports.[32] Individual case safety reports are submitted to the FDA voluntarily from the public; the FAERS relies on health care professionals, patients, caregivers, and others to report adverse events voluntarily either to the product's manufacturer, which will subsequently report them to the FDA according to regulations, or to the FDA directly. The informatic structure of the database adheres to the international safety reporting guidance issued by the International Council on Harmonisation[33] and are compliant with the Health Insurance Portability and Accountability Act Privacy Rule.[34] The advantage of the FAERS is the ability to detect rare and serious adverse events, such as SJS; although, as a passive form of surveillance, there are limitations to the FAERS, which include underreporting, duplicate reports, an inability to calculate the incidence of an adverse event, and variable data quality. Notwithstanding these limitations, the FAERS remains a primary and vital source of new safety information in postmarketing surveillance.[35]

Reported adverse events and medication errors are coded to terms in the Medical Dictionary for Regulatory Activities (MedDRA) terminology. The MedDRA provides a clinically validated, multilingual resource that provides standard terminology for adverse event reporting that can be used throughout the drug's life cycle to report adverse events and allow the retrieval of reports at varying levels of granularity.[36] The MedDRA is routinely updated to keep the MedDRA terms current. Although the MedDRA allows for standardization, increased specificity by including nonadverse event terms (eg, medical history, social history, surgical procedures, diagnostic testing), and flexibility in report retrieval, the use of the MedDRA

may also contribute to signal dilution due to the number of terms available.[37] To address some limitations, Standardized MedDRA Queries were created to facilitate the retrieval of cases using grouped search terms that may not be related in its hierarchical structure. For example, Standardized MedDRA Queries were developed for drug reaction and eosinophilia and systemic symptoms as well as severe cutaneous adverse reactions.[38] Despite its limitations, the MedDRA is widely used across regulatory agencies and industry to conduct pharmacovigilance.

Medical literature

The body of published medical literature also serves as an important source for postmarketing safety signals. In contrast with FAERS, published cases are fewer in number, but are often higher in quality given the peer review process. Published case reports tend to include more clinical details to support the confirmation of a particular adverse event and allow a more thorough causality assessment. For example, in a case of SJS associated with a drug, published case reports tend to include details such as skin biopsy results, allergy testing, treatment management, and drug exposure history, according to expert diagnostic and management guidelines.[39,40] The Divisions of Pharmacovigilance staff use automated alerts available in the major biomedical literature databases (eg, PubMed, Embase) to monitor for adverse event reports for a given drug.

FAERS data mining and reporting rates

In addition to monitoring the FAERS and the medical literature for safety signals, the FDA also conducts data mining of the FAERS data.[35] Given the exponentially increasing size of the FAERS database, data mining supports the detection of safety signals in a systematic manner through disproportionality analysis. In this case, an increased proportion of a specific adverse event–drug combination compared with the adverse event reported with all other drugs may indicate a potential safety signal. To generate this safety signal hypotheses for a potential adverse event–drug combination, the FDA can search the FAERS database for a specific adverse event, such as SJS, and generate a test statistical of the adverse event for a particular drug. For example, the proportional reporting ratio (PRR) for SJS and drug X can be calculated by taking the proportion of SJS reports for drug X and dividing it by the proportion of SJS reports for all other drugs in the FAERS database. Using the example data in **Table 2**, the PRR for SJS and drug X can be calculated, where $PRR = [(A/A + B)/(C/C + D)]$. In this example, the PRR is 5.9 and, because the PRR is greater than 1, would be interpreted as FAERS reporting for SJS and drug X is 5.9 times more frequent than what is observed for SJS and all other drugs in the FAERS. This outcome suggests but does not confirm a possible safety signal; the SJS–drug X combination would need to be further evaluated as a potential safety signal.

Although the incidence of an adverse event with a drug cannot be calculated using the FAERS data, reporting rates (sometimes referred to as reporting ratios) of an adverse event with a drug may provide context for a specific adverse event–drug combination, such as the potential population at risk. The reporting rate can be calculated by dividing the number of US cases reported for the adverse event by an estimate of the drug's use in a period of time (eg, number of US prescriptions dispensed). Like data mining results, reporting rates may suggest a potential safety signal and is not confirmation of a signal. As an example, if the reporting rate for SJS and drug X exceeds the expected background rate of SJS in the general population (ie, 1–7 cases per million people), then drug X may be a potential cause of the excess cases reported.

Of note, the underlying limitations of the data used to calculate disproportionality measures and reporting rates must be considered in interpreting these analyses.

Sentinel

Sentinel is the FDA CDER's drug safety surveillance system using national electronic health care data. The FDA Sentinel Initiative was launched in response to the FDA Amendments Act of 2007 and started with the Mini-Sentinel Pilot before transitioning to the full Sentinel System in September 2014.[41] In 2016, the FDA established the Active Postmarket Risk Identification and Analysis System, integrating the Sentinel System into the FDA's regulatory programs.[42] Analyses from the Active Postmarket Risk Identification and Analysis system have provided significant contributions to the evaluations of safety issues including for CADRs. For example, the system has been used to evaluate occurrence of nonmelanoma skin cancer after hydrochlorothiazide use[43] and resulted

in updating the drug label to include the following language.

Nonmelanoma skin cancer Hydrochlorothiazide is associated with an increased risk of nonmelanoma skin cancer. In a study conducted in the Sentinel System, increased risk was predominantly for squamous cell carcinoma and in white patients taking large cumulative doses. The increased risk for squamous cell carcinoma in the overall population was approximately 1 additional case per 16,000 patients per year, and for white patients taking a cumulative dose of >50,000 mg the risk increase was approximately 1 additional SCC case for every 6,700 patients per year.[44]

Safety Signal Evaluation

Once a signal is identified, a multidisciplinary safety team conducts a comprehensive review of the available evidence related to the adverse event–drug combination. Available data sources include preclinical data, literature, other safety databases, clinical trials and studies from preapproval development programs, epidemiologic studies, product use data, and reporting rates (or ratios); all available data are considered in the formulation of conclusions regarding the causal association between a suspect drug and an adverse event.[21,22,26] The safety team includes safety evaluators, medical officers, and epidemiologists, as well as any other subject matter experts that can provide additional expertise relevant to the specific adverse event–drug combination, such as pharmacogenetic aspects.

For CADRs, given the rarity of serious cutaneous reactions like SJS/TEN, case data often are critical to signal evaluation. To develop case-level data, the safety team develops a case series using selection criteria to query the FAERS database broadly and identify potential individual cases. The selection criteria includes "specific combinations of signs, symptoms, and test results" based on "the medical literature and current expert clinical guidelines."[26] Each FAERS report is individually screened to determine if the report includes the adverse event of interest and sufficient information to allow for an assessment of drug

Table 2
Disproportionality analysis example[a]: FAERS SJS reporting with drug X and all other drugs in the FAERS database

	SJS	All other events in the FAERS
Reports for drug X	10 (A)	500 (B)
Reports for all other drugs	50 (C)	15,000 (D)

[a] Not real data from the FAERS; values chosen to illustrate potential case.

causality. If the FAERS report lacks information, the safety evaluator may contact the reporter to obtain the additional information needed. The identified FAERS reports are reviewed against the selection criteria for inclusion in the case series and duplicate reports are screened out. This process is repeated for published case reports in the medical literature. The selected, deduplicated case reports comprise the case series that then undergoes assessment for causal association.

The focus of causal association is the evaluation of relatedness between the adverse event and the reported drug exposure of the individual. Aspects considered by the safety evaluator include:[26]

(1) Chronologic data (eg, plausible temporal sequence, dechallenge, rechallenge)
(2) Precedents (eg, similar adverse events with the same product or related products)
(3) Biological or pharmacologic plausibility (eg, toxic drug concentration in body fluid, occurrence of a recognized pharmacodynamic phenomenon)
(4) Information quality, and
(5) Alternative etiologies (eg, concurrent diseases or conditions, concomitant medications).

In general, the information from the FAERS and published case reports cannot provide definitive evidence of causal association between an adverse event and drug. "However, a well-documented case of a rare adverse event, that is usually drug-related, or a well-documented report of positive rechallenge can be sufficient to strongly suggest or even establish a causal association."[26] Of note to dermatologists, the determination for a causal association between a drug and the adverse event of SJS/TEN can be made based on a single, well-documented case report; thus, it is important for dermatologists to report these clinical observations, either to the FDA or via publication.

The safety signal evaluation also evaluates the case series cumulatively, reviewing the summary of clinical characteristics (eg, age, sex, dosage) for patterns or trends and causal assessments at the drug–adverse event level (eg, precedents, biological or pharmacologic plausibility).[26] In addition, if possible and depending on the risk prioritization of the adverse event–drug combination, drug use, reporting rates (or ratios), and review of epidemiologic studies (ie, the Sentinel System, review of published epidemiologic studies) are integrated into the safety signal evaluation. At the conclusion of the evaluation, a determination is made regarding the adverse event–drug association based on the strength of evidence reviewed from all available information.

Regulatory Action Based on the Safety Signal Evaluation

After completion of the evaluation, a multidisciplinary team within the CDER determines if regulatory actions are needed to ensure continued safe use of the drug.[45] Depending on the potential impact to the public health, the actions can include modifying the drug labeling to reflect the new information, issuing a drug safety communication to the public, requiring the applicant conduct a postmarketing study to better characterize the risk, and requiring or updating an approved risk evaluation and mitigation strategy to minimize the identified risk.

Communication of a Newly Identified Safety Risk

Drug labeling

A drug's FDA-approved labeling is the primary information source of a drug's safety and efficacy. The labeling summarizes for the prescriber the evidenced-based information that is essential for the safe and effective use of the drug. The FDA can require applicants to modify the currently approved labeling to include new safety-related information.[46] The structure and content of the labeling is defined in regulation; the FDA has published several guidances describing the process of safety-related labeling changes and how to communicate risks according to the degree of potential impact.[47–50] **Table 3** includes examples of labeling language used to inform health care providers of the risk of SJS/TEN.

Communications

The FDA also uses other forms of communication to disseminate newly identified safety risks to the public. The Drug Safety Communication is one tool used to communicate emerging safety issues that may potentially lead to serious or life-threatening events; Drug Safety Communications generally convey a summary of the data reviewed by the FDA along with recommended actions for health care providers and patients, if appropriate to the risk.[50,26] In addition, the FDA can require the applicant to issue "Dear Healthcare Provider" letters describing significant hazards to safety, announce important changes to drug labeling, or emphasize corrections in prescription drug advertising and drug labeling.[50,26] In certain cases, the FDA can also create and include on its web site Consumer Updates describing safety information for consumers. The FDA-identified safety risks are also published in the biomedical literature. **Table 4** highlights examples of these types of communications relevant to the practice of dermatology.[11,12,51–55]

Table 3
Examplesᵃ of labeling language that describes the risk of serious skin reactions with the approved drug's use

Labeling Section	Language
Boxed Warning	*WARNING: SERIOUS SKIN RASHES* LAMICTAL XR can cause serious rashes requiring hospitalization and discontinuation of treatment. The incidence of these rashes, which have included Stevens–Johnson syndrome, is approximately 0.8% (8 per 1000) in pediatric patients (aged 2–16 years) receiving immediate-release lamotrigine as adjunctive therapy for epilepsy and 0.3% (3 per 1000) in adults on adjunctive therapy for epilepsy. In a prospectively followed cohort of 1983 pediatric patients (aged 2–16 years) with epilepsy taking adjunctive immediate-release lamotrigine, there was 1 rash-related death. LAMICTAL XR is not approved for patients younger than 13 years. In worldwide postmarketing experience, rare cases of toxic epidermal necrolysis and/or rash-related death have been reported in adult and pediatric patients, but their numbers are too few to permit a precise estimate of the rate. The risk of serious rash caused by treatment with LAMICTAL XR is not expected to differ from that with immediate-release lamotrigine. However, the relatively limited treatment experience with LAMICTAL XR makes it difficult to characterize the frequency and risk of serious rashes caused by treatment with LAMICTAL XR. Other than age, there are as yet no factors identified that are known to predict the risk of occurrence or the severity of rash caused by LAMICTAL XR. There are suggestions, yet to be proven, that the risk of rash may also be increased by (1) coadministration of LAMICTAL XR with valproate (includes valproic acid and divalproex sodium), (2) exceeding the recommended initial dose of LAMICTAL XR, or (3) exceeding the recommended dose escalation for LAMICTAL XR. However, cases have occurred in the absence of these factors. Nearly all cases of life-threatening rashes caused by immediate-release lamotrigine have occurred within 2–8 weeks of treatment initiation. However, isolated cases have occurred after prolonged treatment (e.g., 6 months). Accordingly, duration of therapy cannot be relied upon as means to predict the potential risk heralded by the first appearance of a rash. Although benign rashes are also caused by LAMICTAL XR, it is not possible to predict reliably which rashes will prove to be serious or life threatening. Accordingly, LAMICTAL XR should ordinarily be discontinued at the first sign of rash, unless the rash is clearly not drug related. Discontinuation of treatment may not prevent a rash from becoming life threatening or permanently disabling or disfiguring *[see Warnings and Precautions (5.1)]*.
Section 4: Contraindications	REYATAZ is contraindicated: · in patients with previously demonstrated clinically significant hypersensitivity (eg, Stevens–Johnson syndrome, erythema multiforme, or toxic skin eruptions) to any of the components of REYATAZ capsules or REYATAZ oral powder *[see Warnings and Precautions (5.2)]*.

(continued on next page)

Table 3 (continued)	
Labeling Section	**Language**
Section 5: Warnings and Precautions	**Serious Skin Reactions** Serious skin reactions have occurred following treatment with Celebrex, including erythema multiforme, exfoliative dermatitis, Stevens–Johnson Syndrome (SJS), toxic epidermal necrolysis (TEN), drug reaction with eosinophilia and systemic symptoms (DRESS), and acute generalized exanthematous pustulosis (AGEP). These serious events may occur without warning and can be fatal.
	Inform patients about the signs and symptoms of serious skin reactions, and to discontinue the use of CELEBREX at the first appearance of skin rash or any other sign of hypersensitivity. CELEBREX is contraindicated in patients with previous serious skin reactions to NSAIDs [*see Contraindications (4)*].
Section 6: Adverse Reactions	6.2 Postmarketing experience
	The following additional adverse reactions have been identified during post-approval use of ERLEADA. Because these reactions are reported voluntarily from a population of uncertain size, it is not always possible to reliably estimate the frequency or establish a causal relationship to drug exposure. . .
	Skin and subcutaneous tissue disorders: Stevens–Johnson syndrome/toxic epidermal necrolysis

[a] Language obtained from labels of different applications available on https://www.accessdata.fda.gov/scripts/cder/daf/.

The Role of Dermatologists in Postmarketing Surveillance

The American Medical Association (AMA) Code of Medical Ethics (Code) describes the values physicians embody as members of the medical profession and is based on the Hippocratic oath to "relieve suffering and promote well-being in a relationship of fidelity with the patient."[56] The AMA code includes Opinions of the AMA Council on Ethical and Judicial Affairs to provide guidance to the medical profession, of any specialty, on the essentials of ethical behavior.[57] Opinion 8.8 (Required Reporting of Adverse Events) was updated in 2016 by the AMA House of Delegates and states:[58]

Physicians' professional commitment to advance scientific knowledge and make relevant information available to patients, colleagues, and the public carries with it the responsibility to report suspected adverse events resulting from the use of a drug or medical device. As professionals who prescribe and monitor the use of drugs and medical devices, physicians are best positioned to observe and communicate about adverse events. A physician who suspects that an adverse reaction to a drug or medical device has occurred has an ethical responsibility to:

(a) Communicate that information to the professional community through established reporting mechanisms.
(b) Promptly report serious adverse events requiring hospitalization, death, or medical or surgical intervention to the appropriate regulatory agency.

More recently, in the *British Journal of Dermatology*, an editorial by Garcia-Doval and colleagues[59] called on article authors whose submissions describe adverse events to report the case to the available pharmacovigilance systems. In addition, the authors conclude stating that the *British Journal of Dermatology* will work to ensure that published case reports include the relevant details to enhance its usefulness in post-marketing surveillance as a part of the journal's commitment to drug safety.[59]

Spontaneous reporting is inherently subject to reporting bias given its voluntary nature.[10,66] Physicians have been found to be the least likely of the health care professionals evaluated to report ADRs.[64] In one study, the attitudes of physicians toward adverse reaction reporting were summarized as:[60,61]

"I am unsure how to report an ADR."

Table 4
Examples of FDA communications relevant to dermatologists

Type of Communication	Title of Communication
Drug Safety Communication	FDA Drug Safety Communication: FDA warns about rare but serious skin reactions with mental health drug olanzapine (Zyprexa, Zyprexa Zydis, Zyprexa Relprevv, and Symbyax). FDA Drug Safety Communication for Tumor Necrosis Factors (TNF) Blockers, Azathioprine & Mercaptopurine.
Dear Healthcare Provider Letter	"Dear Doctor" letter from Hoffmann–LaRoche (February 26, 1998) on the inclusion of "psychiatric disorders" into the warning section of labeling.
Consumer update	Do not use: black salve is dangerous and called by many names.
Publication	Thambi L, Konkel K, Diak I-L, Reyes M, McCulley L. Cosmetic disfigurement from black salve. Drugs & Therapy Perspectives. 2020;36(11):526–528. Cheng C, La Grenade L, Diak IL, Brinker A, Levin RL. Chemical Leukoderma Associated with Methylphenidate Transdermal System: Data From the US FDA Adverse Event Reporting System. J Pediatr. 2017;180:241–246. Kothary N, Diak IL, Brinker A, Bezabeh S, Avigan M, Dal Pan G. Progressive multifocal leukoencephalopathy associated with efalizumab use in psoriasis patients. J Am Acad Dermatol. 2011;65(3):546–551.

"I may appear foolish if I report a suspected ADR."
"I may expose myself to legal liability by reporting an ADR."
"I am too busy to report ADRs."
"I am reluctant to admit that I caused harm."
"I would rather collect cases and publish them."
"Only safe drugs are marketed."

The AMA Code Opinion on Required Reporting of Adverse Events addresses physician reluctance to report stating physicians "need not be certain that there is such an event or even that there is a reasonable likelihood of a causal relationship, to suspect that an adverse event has occurred."[57] MedWatch, as described by the FDA Commissioner at the time, was designed to encourage "health care professionals to regard reporting as a fundamental professional and public health responsibility."[25] To facilitate reporting, MedWatch allows submission of cases through an online form, but also provides a downloadable form for submission; the online form supports submission of images, which can be helpful for cutaneous adverse reaction cases. **Box 1** summarizes the options for submitting cases to MedWatch. Although the minimum information required to complete a report include 4 data points (ie, the patient, adverse event, suspect drug, and reporter name), a thorough report takes approximately 15 to 20 minutes to complete.[62] Because it is not practical to submit every case, several authors have recommended reporting suspected ADRs that are serious or unexpected, from newly approved drugs (within 3 years of approval), and are considered high risk by regulatory agencies.[63–65] During a busy clinic or hospital day, finding the time to report may pose a challenge to timely, complete submissions. To address this, some health organizations allow for an operationalized approach leveraging pharmacists and nurses, or a drug safety officer, to support the routine submission of ADR reports.[62,63]

The FAERS is limited by the variability and lack of information included in reports. Improving the usefulness of spontaneous reporting systems

Box 1
Options for submitting cases to FDA's MedWatch program

Online: MedWatch Website	www.fda.gov/medwatch/report.htm
Phone (toll-free)	1–800-FDA (332)-1088
Fax (toll-free)	1–800-FDA(332)-0178

includes increasing reporting of suspected ADRs as well as improving the quality of the reports submitted. Notably, capturing a small proportion of ADRs through reporting may still have a large impact if those reports contain the necessary information to make an adequate assessment of causal association.[65,66] In the case of rare adverse events, such as SJS/TEN, the infrequent occurrence of the adverse event compounds the limitations of underreporting and lack of details in poor quality reports. Several guidelines exist to ensure that case reports include the necessary information to make an assessment of the adverse event-drug association.[67] Specific to dermatology, the National Institutes of Health Working Group developed a validated case report form for SJS/TEN through a consensus process identifying the elements to include in a standardized case report form; the form does not include a specific causality assessment tool, but serves to provide the necessary information to aid in the diagnosis for a condition where no diagnostic criteria exist.[68]

As articulated by Raschi and colleagues,[69,70] dermatology is experiencing an increase in documented drug-induced skin toxicities, as well as an increase in the use of biologics to treat skin disease, which may have serious noncutaneous adverse reactions. Dermatologists, at the front line of making these clinical observations, are poised to identify new drug safety information that is relevant for improving the public's health. The submission of high-quality case reports, either through postmarketing surveillance systems or published in the literature, can provide valuable clinical data to drug safety regulators. Timely and informative case reports are particularly helpful in informing a drug's safety profile and may lead to updates in the drug's labeling, ultimately improving patient safety and health care provider awareness of safety risks.

SUMMARY

Dermatologists should become more familiar with the regulatory reporting processes for ensuring the continued safe use of approved drugs because of the increase in new drugs approved for dermatologic conditions, approvals for novel drugs with unique mechanisms indicated for nondermatologic conditions where a dermatologist may be consulted for drug-induced adverse events, the common occurrence of CADR, and the rarity of Severe Cutaneous Adverse Reactions. Because dermatologists play a key role in differentiating different types of CADR and in identifying the likely culprit drug in the clinical setting, dermatologists can have a large impact on patient safety through spontaneous reporting of suspected adverse event-drug combinations to the FDA.

CLINICS CARE POINTS

- The drug labeling is a current and comprehensive summary of the safety and efficacy information reviewed by the FDA for approved drugs marketed in the United States.
- The voluntary reporting of observed adverse events with use of drugs enhances the postmarketing surveillance by the FDA, particularly if necessary details are included according to reporting guidelines.
- Dermatologists are positioned to identify the association between a drug and a cutaneous adverse reaction, particularly for uncommon reactions like SJS/TEN, and can aid in signal detection by submitting reports to the FAERS using MedWatch.

DISCLOSURE

This publication reflects the views of the authors and do not necessarily represent the FDA's views or policies.

REFERENCES

1. U.S. Food and Drug Administration. Center for drug evaluation and research web site. Available at: https://www.fda.gov/about-fda/fda-organization/center-drug-evaluation-and-research-cder. Accessed March 20, 2021.
2. A conversation about the FDA and drug regulation with Janet Woodcock, MD, deputy FDA commissioner for operations. Food and Drug Administration Web site. Available at: https://web.archive.org/web/20151228230624/http://www.fda.gov:80/Drugs/ResourcesForYou/Consumers/ucm143467.htm. Accessed March 20, 2021.
3. U.S. Food and Drug Administration. Guidance for industry: development and use of risk minimization action plans. U.S. Department of Health and Human Services; 2005. Available at: https://www.fda.gov/RegulatoryInformation/Guidances/default.htm. Accessed March 7, 2021.
4. U.S. Food and Drug Administration. Guidance for industry: good pharmacovigilance practice and pharmacoepidemiologic assessment. U.S. Department of Health and Human Services; 2005. Available at: https://www.fda.gov/RegulatoryInformation/Guidances/default.htm. Accessed March 7, 2021.

5. Svensson CK, Cowen EW, Gaspari AA. Cutaneous drug reactions. Pharmacol Rev 2001;53(3):357–79.

6. Naldi L, Crotti S. Epidemiology of cutaneous drug-induced reactions. G Ital Dermatol Venereol 2014; 149(2):207–18.

7. Bigby M, Jick S, Jick H, et al. Drug-induced cutaneous reactions. A report from the Boston Collaborative Drug Surveillance Program on 15,438 consecutive inpatients, 1975 to 1982. JAMA 1986; 256(24):3358–63.

8. Hsu DY, Brieva J, Silverberg NB, et al. Morbidity and Mortality of Stevens-Johnson Syndrome and Toxic Epidermal Necrolysis in United States Adults. J Invest Dermatol 2016;136(7):1387–97.

9. Brewer T, Colditz GA. Postmarketing surveillance and adverse drug reactions: current perspectives and future needs. JAMA 1999;281(9):824–9.

10. Dal Pan GJ, Lindquist M, Gelperin K. Postmarketing spontaneous pharmacovigilance reporting systems. Pharmacoepidemiology 2019;165–201.

11. Kothary N, Diak IL, Brinker A, et al. Progressive multifocal leukoencephalopathy associated with efalizumab use in psoriasis patients. J Am Acad Dermatol 2011;65(3):546–51.

12. Cheng C, La Grenade L, Diak IL, et al. Chemical leukoderma associated with methylphenidate transdermal system: data from the US Food and Drug Administration Adverse Event Reporting System. J Pediatr 2017;180:241–6.

13. Asfour L, Yiu ZZN, Warren RB. How is safety of dermatology drugs assessed: trials, registries, and spontaneous reporting. Expert Opin Drug Saf 2020;19(4):449–57.

14. Macklis PC, Dulmage B, Evans B, et al. Cutaneous adverse events in newly approved FDA non-cancer drugs: a systematic review. Drugs R D 2020;20(3):171–87.

15. Rosen AC, Balagula Y, Raisch DW, et al. Life-threatening dermatologic adverse events in oncology. Anticancer Drugs. 2014;25(2):225–34.

16. Ng CY, Chen C-B, Wu M-Y, et al. Anticancer drugs induced severe adverse cutaneous drug reactions: an updated review on the risks associated with anticancer targeted therapy or immunotherapies. J Immunol Res 2018;2018:5376476.

17. Drake LA, Dinehart SM, Farmer ER, et al. Guidelines of care for cutaneous adverse drug reactions. American Academy of Dermatology. J Am Acad Dermatol 1996;35(3 Pt 1):458–61.

18. FDA@Glossary. Food and drug administration Web site. Available at: https://www.accessdata.fda.gov/scripts/cder/daf/index.cfm?event=glossary.page. Accessed on March 21, 2021.

19. 21CFR1.3 Definitions. April 2020. CFR - Code of Federal Regulations Title 21 (fda.gov). Accessed on April 12, 2021.

20. World Health Organization - Uppsala Monitoring Centre. Glossary of Pharmacovigilance terms. Available at: https://www.who-umc.org/global-pharmacovigilance/publications/glossary/. Accessed March 7, 2021.

21. Lester J, Neyarapally GA, Lipowski E, et al. Evaluation of FDA safety-related drug label changes in 2010. Pharmacoepidemiol Drug Saf 2013;22(3):302–5.

22. Ishiguro C, Hall M, Neyarapally GA, et al. Post-market drug safety evidence sources: an analysis of FDA drug safety communications. Pharmacoepidemiol Drug Saf 2012;21(10):1134–6.

23. 21CFR314.80 Postmarketing reporting of adverse drug experiences. 2019. Available at: https://www.accessdata.fda.gov/scripts/cdrh/cfdocs/cfcfr/CFRSearch.cfm?fr=314.80. Accessed on March 7, 2021.

24. Milestones of drug regulation in the United. States. Food and Drug Administration Web site. Available at: https://www.fda.gov/about-fda/history-fdas-centers-and-offices/center-drug-evaluation-and-research-history. Accessed March 20, 2021.

25. Kessler DA, Natanblut S, Kennedy D, et al. Introducing MEDWatch: a new approach to reporting medication and device adverse effects and product problems. JAMA 1993;269(21):2765–8.

26. U.S. Food and Drug Administration. Best Practices in Drug and Biological Product Postmarket Safety Surveillance for FDA Staff. Guidance Draft: 2019;. https://www.fda.gov/media/130216/download. [Accessed 21 March 2021].

27. Food, Drug & cosmetics act. Available at: http://www.gpo.gov/fdsys/pkg/USCODE-2010-title21/html/USCODE-2010-title21-chap9-subchapV-partA-sec355.htm. Accessed March 31, 2021.

28. Center for Drug Evaluation and Research: CDER. Food and drug administration Web site. Available at: https://www.fda.gov/about-fda/fda-organization/center-drug-evaluation-and-research-cder. Accessed March 12, 2021.

29. CDER office of surveillance and epidemiology. Food and drug administration web site. Available at: https://www.fda.gov/about-fda/center-drug-evaluation-and-research-cder/cder-office-surveillance-and-epidemiology. Accessed March 12, 2021.

30. Office of surveillance and epidemiology (OSE) – divisions. Available at: https://www.fda.gov/about-fda/center-drug-evaluation-and-research-cder/office-surveillance-and-epidemiology-ose-divisions. Accessed on March 20, 2021.

31. Importation of prescription drugs, final rule. Available at: Importation of Prescription Final Rule. Accessed March 31, 2021.

32. FDA adverse event reporting system public dashboard. FDA web site. Available at: https://www.fda.gov/drugs/questions-and-answers-fdas-adverse-

event-reporting-system-faers/fda-adverse-event-reporting-system-faers-public-dashboard. Accessed on March 20, 2021.

33. U.S. Food and Drug Administration. Guidance for industry: E2B(R3) electronic transmission of individual case safety reports (ICSRs) implementation guide – data elements and message specification. U.S. Department of Health and Human Services; 2014. Available at: https://www.fda.gov/Regulatory Information/Guidances/default.htm. Accessed March 20, 2021.

34. HIPAA compliance for reporters to FDA MedWatch. FDA web Site. Available at: https://www.fda.gov/safety/reporting-serious-problems-fda/hipaa-compliance-reporters-fda-medwatch#:~:text=You%20can%20continue%20to%20make,event%20reporting%20in%20any%20way. Accessed March 20, 2021.

35. Jones SC, Kortepeter C, Brinker AD. Postmarketing surveillance of drug-induced liver injury. In: Chen M, Will Y, editors. Drug-induced liver toxicity. Methods in pharmacology and toxicology. New York: Humana; 2018. https://doi.org/10.1007/978-1-4939-7677-5_22. Available at:.

36. Medical Dictionary for Regulatory Activities (MedDRA). MedDRA Website. Available at: https://www.meddra.org/. Accessed March 31, 2021.

37. Mozzicato P. MedDRA. Pharm Med 2009;23(2):65–75.

38. List of SMQ Topics (as of 1 September 2020). MedDRA Web site. Available at: https://www.meddra.org/standardised-meddra-queries. Accessed on March 21, 2021.

39. Dodiuk-Gad RP, Chung WH, Valeyrie-Allanore L, et al. Stevens-Johnson syndrome and toxic epidermal necrolysis: an update. Am J Clin Dermatol 2015;16(6):475–93.

40. Shah RR. Importance of Publishing Adverse Drug Reaction Case Reports: Promoting Public Health and Advancing Pharmacology and Therapeutics. Drug Saf - Case Rep 2017;11(4). https://doi.org/10.1007/s40800-017-0053-0.

41. FDA's Sentinel Initiative. Food and Drug Administration Web site. Available at: https://www.fda.gov/safety/fdas-sentinel-initiative. Accessed on March 21, 2021.

42. About the food and drug administration sentinel initiative. Sentinel web site. Available at: https://www.sentinelinitiative.org/. Accessed on March 21, 2021.

43. Eworuke E, Haug N, Bradley M, et al. Risk of nonmelanoma skin cancer in association with use of hydrochlorothiazide-containing products in the United States. JNCI Cancer Spectr 2021;5(2): pkab009.

44. Drugs@FDA. Food and Drug Administration Website. Available at: https://www.accessdata.fda.gov/scripts/cder/daf/. Accessed March 31, 2021.

45. Chamberlain C, Kortepeter C, Muñoz M. Chapter 27: Clinical analysis of adverse drug reactions. In: Fotis M, Budris W, editors. Principles of clinical pharmacology. Elsevier; 2012. p. 455–65.

46. Section 505(o)(4) of the FD&C Act. FD&C Act Chapter V: Drugs and Devices | FDA. Accessed March 31, 20 21.

47. Food and Drug Administration. Guidance for industry: safety labeling changes — implementation of section 505(o)(4) of the FD&C Act. U.S. Department of Health and Human Services; 2013. Available at: https://www.fda.gov/RegulatoryInformation/Guidances/default.htm. Accessed March 21, 2021.

48. Food and Drug Administration. Guidance for industry: adverse reactions section of labeling for human prescription drug and biological products — content and format. U.S. Department of Health and Human Services; 2006. Available at: https://www.fda.gov/RegulatoryInformation/Guidances/default.htm. Accessed March 21, 2021.

49. Food and Drug Administration. Guidance for industry: warnings and precautions, contraindications, and boxed warning sections of labeling for human prescription drug and biological products — content and format. U.S. Department of Health and Human Services; 2011. Available at: https://www.fda.gov/RegulatoryInformation/Guidances/default.htm. Accessed March 21, 2021.

50. Food and Drug Administration. Guidance: drug safety information – FDA's communication to the public. U.S. Department of Health and Human Services; 2012. Available at: https://www.fda.gov/RegulatoryInformation/Guidances/default.htm. Accessed March 21, 2021.

51. FDA drug safety communication for tumor necrosis factors (TNF) blockers, azathioprine & mercaptopurine. Prescribers' Digital Reference Web site. Available at: https://m.pdr.net/fda-drug-safety-communication/remicade?druglabelid=263&id=8846. Accessed on March 21, 2021.

52. FDA Drug Safety Communication: FDA warns about rare but serious skin reactions with mental health drug olanzapine (Zyprexa, Zyprexa Zydis, Zyprexa Relprevv, and Symbyax). Food and Drug Administration Web site. Available at: https://www.fda.gov/drugs/drug-safety-and-availability/fda-drug-safety-communication-fda-warns-about-rare-serious-skin-reactions-mental-health-drug. Accessed on March 21, 2021.

53. Do not use: black salve is dangerous and called by many names. Food and Drug Administration Web site. Published October 13, 2020. Accessed on March 12, 2021.

54. Maddin S. FDA Warning about Isotretinoin (Accutane., Roaccutane.) Skin Therapy Letter Web site. Available at: https://www.skintherapyletter.com/

acne/fda-warning-about-isotretinoin-accutane-roaccutane/. Accessed on March 21. 2021.

55. Thambi L, Konkel K, Diak I-L, et al. Cosmetic disfigurement from black salve. Drugs Ther Perspect 2020;36(11):526–8.

56. Why does the medical profession need a code of ethics? American Medical Association Web site. Available at: https://www.ama-assn.org/delivering-care/ethics/why-does-medical-profession-need-code-ethics. Accessed March 22.2021.

57. Code of medical ethics preface & preamble. American Medical Association Web site. Available at: https://www.ama-assn.org/about/publications-newsletters/code-medical-ethics-preface-preamble. Accessed March 22, 2021.

58. Required reporting of adverse events. American Medical Association Web site. Available at: https://www.ama-assn.org/delivering-care/ethics/required-reporting-adverse-events#:~:text=Code%20of%20Medical%20Ethics%20Opinion,a%20drug%20or%20medical%20device. Accessed March 22, 2021.

59. Garcia-Doval I, Segovia E, Hunter H, et al. The value of case reports in pharmacovigilance. Br J Dermatol 2020;183(5):795–6.

60. Inman WH. Attitudes to adverse drug reaction reporting. Br J Clin Pharmacol 1996;41(5):434–5.

61. Abelson MB, Lafond A. Making the Most of FDA's MedWatch. Rev Ophthalmol 2011. Available at: https://www.reviewofophthalmology.com/article/making-the-most-of-fdas-medwatch. Accessed March 20, 2021.

62. MedWatch Online Voluntary Report. Food and Drug Administration Web site. Available at: https://www.accessdata.fda.gov/scripts/medwatch/index.cfm. [Accessed 22 March 2021]. Accessed.

63. ASHP guidelines on adverse drug reaction monitoring and reporting. Am Soc Hosp Pharm 1995;52(4):417–9.

64. Pushkin R, Frassetto L, Tsourounis C, et al. Improving the reporting of adverse drug reactions in the hospital setting. Postgrad Med 2010;122(6):154–64.

65. How to Report Product Problems and Complaints to the FDA. Food and Drug Administration Web site. Available at: https://www.fda.gov/consumers/consumer-updates/how-report-product-problems-and-complaints-fda. Accessed on March 7, 2021.

66. Berniker JS. Spontaneous reporting systems: achieving less spontaneity and more reporting. 2001.

67. Aronson JK. Case reports as evidence in pharmacovigilance. In: Mann's pharmacovigilance.2014:121-137.

68. Maverakis E, Wang EA, Shinkai K, et al. Stevens-Johnson syndrome and toxic epidermal necrolysis standard reporting and evaluation guidelines: results of a National Institutes of Health Working Group. JAMA Dermatol 2017;153(6):587–92.

69. Raschi E, La Placa M, Poluzzi E, et al. The value of case reports and spontaneous reporting systems for pharmacovigilance and clinical practice. Br J Dermatol 2021;184(3):581–3.

70. Landow Laurence. Monitoring Adverse Drug Events: The Food and Drug Administration MedWatch Reporting System. Regional Anesthesia & Pain Medicine 1998;23:190–3.

How Does the Food and Drug Administration Approve Topical Generic Drugs Applied to the Skin?

Priyanka Ghosh, PhD*, Sam G. Raney, PhD, Markham C. Luke, MD, PhD

KEYWORDS

- Dermatologic • Locally applied • Topical • Generics • Skin diseases

KEY POINTS

- Topical dermatologic drug products are a multibillion-dollar industry in the United States and are widely used for the treatment of various diseases, such as acne, psoriasis, actinic keratosis, and basal cell carcinoma.[1]
- Topical dermatologic drug products encompass a wide array of dosage forms including solutions, gels, creams, lotions, and ointments, among others.
- The Drug Price Competition and Patent Term Restoration Act of 1984 (Public Law 98–417), informally known as the Hatch-Waxman Amendments, established a pathway for approval of generic drug products, including topical dermatologic products, to enhance patient access to such products.
- Approved generic drug products that are therapeutically equivalent to a preidentified brand name drug product (a reference listed drug) are pharmaceutical equivalents for which bioequivalence has been demonstrated. They are expected to have the same clinical effect and safety profile when administered to patients under the conditions specified in the labeling.
- The types of studies used to evaluate the bioequivalence of such drug products typically depends on the site/mechanism of action of the drug product and the complexity of the dosage form.

INTRODUCTION

Topical dermatologic drug products, that is, drug products that are applied to the outer surface of the skin for treatment of skin diseases, are a vital part of a practicing dermatologist's treatment armamentarium. Pastore and colleagues[2] summarized the historic use of oils, fats, perfumes, creams, and so forth to treat disease conditions and wear as cosmetics. The 1966 publication by Bender and Thom[3] discussed the formulation of an ancient cold cream, which was similar to the cream formulations that are available on the market today. However, despite the similarities with ancient formulations, most of the topical dermatologic drug products that are available on the market today are carefully designed using one or more active therapeutic agents (otherwise known as active ingredients) and inactive ingredients to deliver a specific amount of active ingredient per unit area of the skin. Both the formulation development and manufacturing of topical dermatologic drug products have evolved significantly from the days when Galen's Cerate (Cérat de Galien), a cold cream, was one of the most renowned formulas for a dermatologic drug product.

Office of Research and Standards, Office of Generic Drugs, US Food and Drug Administration, 10903 New Hampshire Avenue, Silver Spring, MD 20993, USA
* Corresponding author.
E-mail address: Priyanka.Ghosh@fda.hhs.gov

Dermatol Clin 40 (2022) 279–287
https://doi.org/10.1016/j.det.2022.02.003
0733-8635/22/Published by Elsevier Inc.

Topical dermatologic drugs are one of several pharmaceutical dosage forms that allow for targeted application of a drug to a localized area of the body. This allows for focused therapeutics that minimize the systemic bioavailability (BA) and potential toxicity of the applied drug. There are some drugs that are applied on the skin, which may have an underlying systemic site of action (either in addition to, or exclusive of, any local skin effect). In other instances, a topical dermatologic drug product may be applied to diseased skin, which may or may not be intact. Some topical products exhibit therapeutic effects that rely on the fact that the diseased or wounded skin is not intact (ie, the rate-limiting barrier to skin permeation, the stratum corneum, is nonexistent or compromised). Yet other topical dermatologic drug products may actually target a localized infestation, which may be exterior to the surface of the skin. Finally, concern for some locally acting drugs' systemic toxicity may prompt the need to assess that formulation's systemic availability.

HISTORY OF TOPICAL DRUG REGULATIONS IN THE UNITED STATES

In 1906, the Pure Food and Drug Act was one of the first laws enacted by Congress to ensure consumer protection against mislabeled vaccines; it led to the development of the US Bureau of Chemistry, which eventually became the US Food and Drug Administration (FDA).[4] Following the sulfanilamide crisis in 1932, Congress enacted the Federal Food, Drug, and Cosmetic Act (FD&C), which gave the FDA authority to veto the marketing of a drug product unless the safety of the product could be established.[5] Between 1938 and 1962, approximately 4500 new drug applications (NDAs) were submitted to the FDA and subsequently marketed in the United States; these drug products included many topical dermatologic products, such as the Kenalog (triamcinolone acetonide) topical ointment, which is indicated for relief of the inflammatory and pruritic manifestations of corticosteroid-responsive dermatoses. Eventually, following the thalidomide tragedy in Europe, the 1962 Kefauver-Harris Amendments to the FD&C Act were enacted, which required premarket approval of all drug products, including topical dermatologic drug products sold in the United States.[6] Most significantly, the 1962 amendments to the FD&C Act led to the requirement for safety and efficacy data using adequate and well-controlled clinical studies to support the approval of a drug product. Drug products that were authorized for marketing at the time (between 1932 and 1968) had to be reviewed by the FDA for efficacy in addition to the previously reviewed safety data. The administrative process that was used to review the effectiveness of such drug products is known as the drug efficacy study implementation.[7] Topical dermatologic drug products, such as the triamcinolone acetonide topical ointment, among others, were reviewed and found to be efficacious under the drug efficacy study implementation program.

In 1984, to enhance patient access through streamlining the approval of therapeutically equivalent generic drug products, Congress enacted the Drug Price Competition and Patent Term Restoration Act,[8] informally known as the Hatch-Waxman Amendments. The amendments to the FD&C Act made it possible for companies to manufacture and obtain FDA approval for generic drug products by submitting an Abbreviated New Drug Application (ANDA) instead of an NDA. Compared with a drug product that is submitted under an NDA, which contains full reports of investigations of safety and effectiveness, a drug product submitted under an ANDA relies on FDA finding that the preidentified reference listed drug (RLD) is safe and effective and generally must show that the generic drug product is among other things, bioequivalent to the corresponding RLD. The Code of Federal Regulations (CFR) Title 21, Part 320 outlines the kind of data that can be used to establish the bioequivalence (BE) of a given generic product. Within the scope of the current review, the goal is to discuss the rigorous methodologies and different types of evidence that are typically used to support the approval of generic topical dermatologic drug products (small molecules). Such evidence is often related to the complexity of the topical dermatologic dosage form involved.

During the last decade, the use of biologics has been widely recognized as one of the major breakthroughs in the treatment of topical dermatologic diseases, such as psoriasis. Biologics are typically complex mixtures that are sourced from humans, animals, or microorganisms, and represent a different class of drugs compared with the chemically synthesized small molecules with known structures. Biologic drug products are submitted for approval under Section 351 of the Public Health Service Act[9] and are beyond the scope of the current review, which focuses exclusively on pathways used to support the approval of small molecules via the ANDA pathway.

COMMONLY USED TOPICAL DERMATOLOGIC DOSAGE FORMS

Topical dermatologic dosage forms, such as Galen's Cerate (Cérat de Galien), a cold cream, and medicated plasters (*emplastra*), which were generally applied to the skin for local conditions, are traced back to Ancient Greek and Chinese civilizations. Currently, numerous topical dermatologic dosage forms outlined in **Fig. 1** are available on the US market. The most commonly used topical dermatologic dosage forms include gels, creams, lotions, ointments, foams, solutions, and others; they are routinely used to treat a wide array of diseases. Some examples include topical dermatologic drug products that contain antiparasitic agents used in the treatment of head lice. These topical products, which include malathion or benzyl alcohol topical lotions, are applied to the scalp and work on an organism that is external to the human body. Antifungal products, such as efinaconazole and tavaborole solutions, are used for the treatment of onychomycosis of the toenail. More commonly, retinoid- and antibiotic-containing products, such as the tretinoin topical gels and creams, tazarotene topical gels and creams, and clindamycin topical gels, are used for the treatment of acne vulgaris; and antibiotic-containing products, such as the metronidazole topical gels and creams, are used for the treatment of rosacea. Topical ointments and creams products containing synthetic vitamin D_3 derivates, such as calcipotriene, are used in the treatment of psoriasis; whereas topical calcineurin inhibitors, such as pimecrolimus, and immunosuppressive

agents, such as tacrolimus, are used for the treatment of atopic dermatitis.

The previously outlined examples illustrate that numerous active ingredients in a wide array of dosage forms are used to treat different skin diseases. The selection of the dosage form is typically driven by the feasibility of formulating the active ingredient in a given dosage form and influenced by factors, such as patient perceptions and ease of use. For example, although an occlusive topical ointment may be preferred for the treatment of atopic dermatitis, a rapidly evaporating gel or cream may be preferred for the treatment of facial acne.

A topical dermatologic dosage form usually contains one or more active ingredients. A 2005 publication briefly outlined a scientifically based, systematic classification of dosage forms for topical drugs.[10] From a technical perspective, a solution is a dosage form where the active ingredient is completely solubilized in the drug product. A topical suspension is a dosage form where the active ingredient is partially suspended in the continuous phase; in such cases the active ingredient is expected to dissolve before it is available for diffusion across the stratum corneum barrier of the skin. Gels are typically manufactured by adding a polymerizing/gelling agent to a mixture of active and inactive ingredients. Both aqueous-based and alcohol-based gels are available on

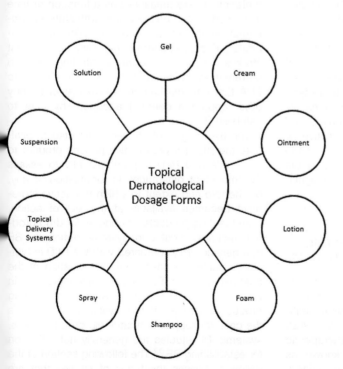

Fig. 1. The 10 most commonly used topical dermatologic dosage forms in the United States.[12]

the US market, and most gels are single-phase systems where the active ingredient is either fully or partially dissolved in the continuous phase. Emulsion-based gels (ie, gels that are manufactured to be biphasic systems) are less common, but such products (eg, diclofenac sodium [emulsion-based] gels) are also available on the US market.[11] Lotions and creams are typically biphasic vehicle (emulsion) dosage forms where the active ingredient is either fully or partially dissolved in one or both phases. An ointment is typically manufactured using either a petrolatum base or polyethylene glycols, where the active ingredient is fully or partially dissolved. Unlike the gels, creams, and lotions that undergo rapid drying (metamorphosis) following application on the surface of the skin, ointments typically tend to form an occlusive film following application and, therefore, are often used in the treatment of diseases involving a compromised barrier function of the stratum corneum, such as atopic dermatitis. Foams and sprays are typically manufactured by either adding a propellent to a solution or emulsion dosage form, or by using an air-spray foam pump. Shampoos are solution or emulsion type formulations that contain surfactants, and these drug products are typically manufactured for treatment of diseases of the scalp, such as seborrheic dermatitis. Lastly, topical delivery systems (also known as patches) are conceptually similar to medicated plasters where the drug is loaded onto an adhesive matrix or hydrogel-based system; the delivery systems are expected to adhere to the skin and deliver drug across the surface area of application over a specific period of time. Note that the discussion related to the most commonly used dosage forms within the current review is focused on dosage forms that are typically used as pharmaceutical interventions for the treatment of skin diseases with limited and controlled exposure to the active and inactive ingredients, compared with using similar dosage forms in cosmetics where the exposure to the components of the dosage form may be significantly higher.

APPROACHES FOR ESTABLISHING THERAPEUTIC EQUIVALENCE OF GENERIC TOPICAL DERMATOLOGIC DRUG PRODUCTS

For a product to be considered therapeutically equivalent to a preidentified brand name drug or RLD, the generic product must be pharmaceutically equivalent and bioequivalent to the RLD. The Approved Drug Products with Therapeutic Equivalence Evaluations (commonly known as the Orange Book)[12] defines a pharmaceutically equivalent drug product as one that contains an identical amount of the same active ingredient, in an identical dosage form, administered by the same route of administration. Approved generic drug products are considered to be therapeutic equivalents to the preidentified RLD if they are pharmaceutical equivalents for which BE has been demonstrated and can be substituted with the full expectation that the substituted product will have the same clinical effect and safety profile as the RLD when administered to patients under the conditions specified in the drug product label. The type of evidence that is typically required for establishing the BE of a generic topical dermatologic product depends on the site/mechanism of action of the drug product and the complexity of the dosage form.

According to 21 CFR 320.24, the following in vivo and in vitro approaches are acceptable for establishing the BE of a drug product: (1) an in vivo test in humans where the concentration of the active ingredient or active moiety, and, when appropriate, its active metabolites, in whole blood, plasma, serum, or other appropriate biologic fluid is measured as a function of time; (2) an in vivo test in humans where the urinary excretion of the active moiety and, when appropriate, its active metabolites, are measured as a function of time; (3) an in vivo test in humans in which an appropriate acute pharmacologic effect of the active moiety, and, when appropriate, its active metabolites, are measured as a function of time if such effect can be measured with sufficient accuracy, sensitivity, and reproducibility; (4) appropriately designed comparative clinical end point studies, for purposes of demonstrating BE; (5) a currently available in vitro test acceptable to FDA that ensures human in vivo BA; or (6) any other approach deemed adequate by FDA to establish BE.

The overall goal of studies conducted to evaluate the BE of a prospective generic product to the predefined RLD is predominantly to assess the impact of differences in formulation, if any, on the rate and extent to which the active ingredient becomes available at the site of action, from the drug products. In general, for drug products that are indicated for systemic action, the BE of a generic drug compared with the RLD is typically established based on an evaluation of the pharmacokinetics (PK) of the active ingredient in the blood (serum/plasma). However, when a drug product is not intended for systemic action, as is the case for topical dermatologic drug products, systemic PK studies are generally not relied on for establishing BE.[13] The following section of the review discusses the types of studies that are typically used for establishing the BE of topical dermatologic dosage forms.

Comparative Clinical End Points Bioequivalence Studies

Historically, a BE study with a comparative clinical end point has routinely been used for establishing the BE of locally acting topical dermatologic products, such as those mentioned previously. Such studies span weeks to months and are usually conducted in a patient population relevant to the indication of the drug product identified within the product labeling. Typically, hundreds to thousands of patients are required to adequately power such a study to demonstrate the BE of a proposed generic product compared with the predefined RLD. Both products are also expected to demonstrate superiority over a placebo formulation in such studies, as a control. Although comparative clinical end point studies have been successfully used for establishing the BE of topical dermatologic dosage forms, such studies are expensive and time consuming (given the large number of patients and the long duration of the study before the comparative clinical end point may be achieved), and may not be the most sensitive or discriminating method for evaluating differences in the BA of an active ingredient from a proposed generic product compared with the predefined RLD.

Pharmacodynamic Bioequivalence Studies

In addition to the comparative clinical end point BE studies, in limited instances, a pharmacodynamic BE study that uses a vasoconstrictor response for corticosteroids has been used for topical dermatologic dosage forms containing glucocorticoids. However, over the last decade, the FDA has systematically invested in research[14] to develop more efficient approaches for evaluating the BE of locally acting topical dermatologic dosage forms. Based on the FDA's current understanding of the complexity of the different topical dermatologic dosage forms, the following approaches can typically be used for establishing the BE of such drug products.

Waiver of In Vivo Bioequivalence Studies for Topical Solutions

The 21 CFR 320.22(b) (3) states that for certain drug products, the in vivo BA or BE of the drug product may be self-evident. To be able to use this waiver, topical solutions that are applied to the skin must contain the same active ingredient at the same concentration and dosage form as the predefined RLD and not contain any inactive ingredient or other change in formulation that may significantly affect the local or systemic availability of the active ingredient.

Characterization-Based Approaches for Topical Gels, Creams, Lotions, and Ointments

The FDA has recently published several product-specific guidances[15] for generic drug development for topical products in which efficient characterization-based approaches have been recommended for establishing BE, as a complement to comparative clinical end point BE studies. In some instances, the comparative in vitro characterization data of the drug products are used to establish the pharmaceutical equivalence of a prospective generic product compared with the predefined RLD, or to gain additional evidence to mitigate the risk of potential failure modes for BE that may be unique to a drug product. In several other instances, efficient characterization-based approaches are recommended as a stand-alone option, offered as an alternative to a comparative clinical end point BE study. From a scientific perspective, the characterization-based approaches are developed such that the methodology is used to design a prospective generic product that is essentially identical to a predefined reference product with respect to the composition and the microstructure of the drug product, and any differences between a prospective generic product and the predefined reference product are similar to what would be expected across multiple batches of the reference product itself.

Currently, efficient characterization-based approaches are used for establishing the BE of prospective generic drug products that contain no difference in inactive ingredients or in other aspects of the formulation relative to the predefined reference product that may significantly affect the local or systemic availability of the active ingredient. For example, if a prospective generic and the predefined reference product are qualitatively (Q1) and quantitatively (Q2) the same, as defined in the guidance for industry ANDA Submissions–Refuse-to-Receive Standards (December 2016), the BE of such a prospective generic product may be established using a characterization-based BE approach. Such formulation sameness of the drug products is expected to mitigate the risk of known failure modes for therapeutic equivalence related to irritation, sensitization, and issues related to interaction of the formulation with the abnormal, diseased anatomy, physiology, and morphology of the skin, which may arise when there are differences in inactive ingredients between a prospective generic product and the corresponding reference product. Additionally, formulation sameness generally ensures that the stability, solubility, and physical state of the active ingredient in the formulation, which can potentially impact the diffusion and partitioning of active ingredient from the drug product into the skin, are identical for the prospective generic and pre-defined reference product. Sameness of formulation may also mitigate the risks associated with differences in contribution of the vehicle toward efficacy of drug products.

In general, as the complexity of the dosage form increases (eg, solution ⇒ gel ⇒ cream), the number of potential failure modes for BE often also increases. Therefore, the precise type of physicochemical and structural (Q3) characterizations that are recommended as a component of the characterization-based approaches is determined rationally based on the nature of the dosage form, and the potential differences in product quality that may impact the therapeutic performance of a given drug product. Such comparative studies typically include the following:

- An evaluation of visual appearance and microstructural characterization (including microscopic images at multiple magnifications) to be able to visualize and identify differences in the microstructure of the prospective generic and reference products, if any.
- Based on the microscopic evaluation, for products that contain suspended active ingredients, comparative evaluation of particle size distribution and polymorphic form of the active ingredient is recommended because differences in the particle size distribution and/or the polymorphic form of the active ingredient can lead to differences in the solubility of the active ingredient in the drug product and/or the rate of dissolution of the suspended active ingredient. Based on Fick's laws of diffusion, soluble drug can diffuse in molecular form across the stratum corneum. Therefore, differences in the amount of solubilized drug or the rate of dissolution of the active ingredient can impact the BA of the active ingredient from the dosage form.
- For a monophasic system, such as a gel, an evaluation of the microstructure of the dosage form using high-resolution microscopy is usually informative to compare the microstructure of such polymeric gel-based systems. However, for biphasic systems, such as the lotions and the creams that were previously described within the review, an evaluation of the globule size distribution of the emulsion is recommended, because differences in

globule size distribution can impact the interaction of the different phases of the dosage form with the skin, especially as the dosage form dries, which in turn can impact the BA of the active ingredient from the dosage form.
- A comparative evaluation of the rheology of the non-Newtonian semisolid formulations is recommended, given that rheologic differences between a prospective generic and the reference product may impact the look and feel of the product and the corresponding patient perception of quality, and the patient acceptance of the product. Additionally, differences in rheologic properties can also lead to differences in the diffusion of the active ingredient within the dosage form and the amount of the active ingredient that is dispensed before application of the drug product. For example, most topical dermatologic drug product labeling recommends that patients should dispense and use a sufficient amount of the drug product to cover the intended treatment area rather than specifying a predetermined amount/dose. Therefore, it is possible that a smaller amount of a less viscous drug product may be used to treat a surface area that would typically require a larger amount of a more viscous drug product. Such potential differences in rheology, if any, can thereby impact the BA of the active ingredient from the drug product in addition to patient perception and therapeutic compliance.
- A comparative evaluation of the specific gravity/density is also used to ensure that the amount of entrapped air that may be introduced in the formulation during manufacturing processes (eg, the homogenization or emulsification steps used during the manufacture of biphasic formulations, or the gelling of single-phase gels) is consistent between the prospective generic and reference product. Differences in the amount of entrapped air also has the potential to impact the amount of drug product/active ingredient that is dispensed and applied to the skin, and thereby the BA from a given drug product.
- A comparative evaluation of pH is recommended to mitigate the risk of potential irritation, which can impact the patient's acceptability of the product and to ensure a similar solubility and stability of the active ingredient in the drug product, especially in situations where the pKa of the active ingredient is similar to the target pH of the drug product. Small differences in pH between a prospective generic product and the corresponding reference product in such instances can lead to

differences in the amount of solubilized active ingredient in the drug product and thereby the BA of the active ingredient from the drug product.

- Additional comparative Q3 tests may include an evaluation of water activity, that is, a comparative evaluation of the amount of unbound/free water molecules in biphasic formulations and/or an evaluation of the drying rate to understand differences, if any, in the metamorphosis of a prospective generic product and the reference product. Such differences in turn could impact the BA of the active ingredient from the drug product.

An in vitro release test (IVRT), which is designed to evaluate the apparent rate of release of the active ingredient from a drug product, is typically recommended to detect differences, if any, in the apparent rate of release of the active ingredient from the prospective generic and reference products, which may arise because of differences in the microstructure of the drug product that may not be detectable using the previously mentioned comparative Q3 characterization. An adequately validated IVRT is sensitive to differences in the rate of release of the active ingredient from the drug product, and thereby, is useful to mitigate potential failure modes for BE that may arise because of differences in manufacturing processes between a prospective generic product and a reference product.

For complex dosage forms, such as biphasic emulsions, a comparative evaluation of the interaction of the drug product with the skin during metamorphosis (drying of the drug product following application to the skin) may be used to evaluate the BA of the active ingredient from a prospective generic product and the corresponding reference product following application of the drug product to the skin. Such studies that involve a comparison of the cutaneous PK of the drug product in vitro, can be conducted using an in vitro model, such as the in vitro permeation test.[16,17]

As previously noted within the review evaluating the systemic BA using a PK study is typically not relevant for locally acting topical dermatologic drug products where the site of action of the drug product is not systemic. However, in limited instances a crossover in vivo study with PK end points may be used to evaluate the rate and extent of systemic availability of the active ingredient in situations where the site and/or mechanism of action of a topically applied drug product may be partially systemic. An example of a product where such studies have been used includes the diclofenac sodium topical (emulsion-based) gel where the perceived site of action of the drug product

is the synovial fluid[18] and the product is indicated for the relief of osteoarthritic pain.

Combination of Multiple In Vivo Studies

In limited instances, a BE study with PK end points and a BE study with comparative clinical end points may be used for certain drug products when there are differences in the formulation between a prospective generic drug product and the corresponding reference product. For example, for the diclofenac sodium topical (emulsion-based) gel, although the drug is detectable in the plasma, there have been speculative concerns that because of the low BA of diclofenac following topical application of the drug product, only a small difference may be observed between systemic levels of diclofenac delivered from the generic and corresponding reference drug products, despite a potentially significant difference in the amounts of diclofenac delivered locally to the site of application. Additionally, because the exact mechanism of action of diclofenac in osteoarthritis is not well understood and the site of action of the drug product is not well defined (believed to be the structures around the joint or in the synovial fluid), a BE study with comparative clinical end point in addition to the BE study with PK end points is used for establishing BE of such drug products.

Therefore, generic topical dermatologic products may use one or more approaches for establishing BE. An in vivo BE approach, which includes a BE study with comparative clinical end point, or an in vivo vasoconstrictor assay for corticosteroid products, may be used by many proposed generic products (irrespective of the differences in formulation with respect to the reference product) because the recommended in vivo studies are expected to mitigate the risks associated with potential failure modes for BE, regardless of the formulation of the test product. However, a characterization-based BE approach may be applicable to a subset of proposed generic products that contain no difference in inactive ingredients or other aspects of the formulation relative to the reference product that may significantly affect the local or systemic availability of the active ingredient. In addition to "no difference" in the formulation, the recommendations within the characterization-based BE approach may include the following studies to support a demonstration of BE, depending on the complexity of the dosage form and the mechanism/site of action of the drug product: comparative Q3 characterization of the test and reference products, a comparative IVRT study, a comparative in vitro permeation test study, and a BE study with PK end points. The types of studies that are recommended by the FDA to systematically mitigate the risks associated with potential failure modes for BE for a specific product are typically outlined within a product-specific guidance.[15] These product-specific guidances, in conjunction with relevant general guidance for industry,[19] are an excellent resource that can be used by the generic industry to develop high-quality generic products in a manner compatible with regulatory expectations. Additionally, such tools as physiologically based modeling and simulation tools are currently being developed to support the characterization-based approaches for establishing BE.

SUMMARY

According to a US Government Accountability Office report,[20] 57% of topical drug products experienced a price increase of more than 100% between 2010 and 2015, with the average price of topical generic drugs being 276% higher by 2015. Therefore, it is critically important to use efficient approaches for establishing the BE of topical dermatologic drug products to be able to increase market competition and to enhance patient access to such products. This current review systematically discusses the complexity of topical dermatologic dosage forms that are available on the US market and are used to treat a wide array of common dermatologic diseases. Current methodologies used for evaluating the equivalence of a prospective generic product involve a systematic and rigorous comparative evaluation of the drug products using one or more studies to ensure that the rate and extent of BA of the active ingredients at or near the site of action is comparable between the prospective generic and corresponding brand name product.

CLINICS CARE POINTS

- Approved generic drug products are expected to have the same clinical effect and safety profile as the brand name drug when administered to patients under the conditions specified in the labeling.
- Current methodologies used for evaluating the equivalence of a prospective generic product involves a systematic and rigorous comparative evaluation of the drug products using one or more studies.
- FDA works to ensure that generic topical dermatologic drug products are easily accessible to prescribers and patients.

DISCLOSURE STATEMENT

The authors have nothing to disclose.
This article reflects the views of the authors and should not be construed to represent FDA views or policies.

REFERENCES

1. Gaille B. 23 dermatology industry statistics and trends. BrandonGaille.com. Available at: https://brandongaille.com/23-dermatology-industry-statistics-and-trends/. Accessed August 26, 2021.
2. Pastore MN, Kalia YN, Horstmann M, et al. Transdermal patches: history, development and pharmacology. Br J Pharmacol 2015;172(9):2179–209.
3. Bender GA, Thom RA. Great moments in medicine and pharmacy: a history of medicine and pharmacy in pictures. Detroit, MI: Northwood Institute Press; 1966.
4. Part I: the 1906 Food and Drugs Act and its enforcement. U.S. Food and Drug Administration. Available at: https://www.fda.gov/about-fda/changes-science-law-and-regulatory-authorities/part-i-1906-food-and-drugs-act-and-its-enforcement. Accessed August 26, 2021.
5. Part II: 1938, Food, Drug, Cosmetic Act. U.S. Food and Drug Administration. Available at: https://www.fda.gov/about-fda/changes-science-law-and-regulatory-authorities/part-ii-1938-food-drug-cosmetic-act. Accessed August 26, 2021.
6. Part III: drugs and foods under the 1938 act and its amendments. Available at: https://www.fda.gov/about-fda/changes-science-law-and-regulatory-authorities/part-iii-drugs-and-foods-under-1938-act-and-its-amendments. Accessed October 21, 2021.
7. Center for Drug Evaluation and Research. Drug efficacy study implementation (DESI). U.S. Food and Drug Administration. Available at: https://www.fda.gov/drugs/enforcement-activities-fda/drug-efficacy-study-implementation-desi. Accessed August 26, 2021.
8. Center for Drug Evaluation and Research. Abbreviated new drug application (ANDA): Generics. U.S. Food and Drug Administration. Available at: https://www.fda.gov/drugs/types-applications/abbreviated-new-drug-application-anda. Accessed August 26, 2021.
9. Center for Biologics Evaluation and Research. What are "biologics" questions and answers. U.S. Food and Drug Administration. Available at: https://www.fda.gov/about-fda/center-biologics-evaluation-and-research-cber/what-are-biologics-questions-and-answers. Accessed August 26, 2021.
10. Buhse L, Kolinski R, Westenberger B, et al. Topical drug classification. Int J Pharm 2005;295(1–2):101–12.

11. Tsakalozou E, Babiskin A, Zhao L. Physiologically-based pharmacokinetic modeling to support bio-equivalence and approval of generic products: a case for diclofenac sodium topical gel, 1. CPT Pharmacometrics Syst Pharmacol 2021;10(5):399–411.

12. Center for Drug Evaluation and Research. Approved drug products with therapeutic equivalence evaluations (ORANGE BOOK). U.S. Food and Drug Administration. Available at: https://www.fda.gov/drugs/drug-approvals-and-databases/approved-drug-products-therapeutic-equivalence-evaluations-orange-book. [Accessed 26 August 2021]. Accessed.

13. Raney SG, Franz TJ, Lehman PA, et al. Pharmacokinetics-based approaches for bioequivalence evaluation of topical dermatological drug products. Clin Pharmacokinet 2015;54(11):1095–106.

14. Center for Drug Evaluation and Research. Science & research. U.S. Food and Drug Administration. Available at: https://www.fda.gov/drugs/generic-drugs/science-research. Accessed August 26, 2021.

15. Center for Drug Evaluation and Research. Product-Specific guidances for generic drug development. U.S. Food and Drug Administration. Available at: https://www.fda.gov/drugs/guidances-drugs/product-specific-guidances-generic-drug-development. Accessed August 26, 2021.

16. Franz TJ, Lehman PA, Raney SG. Use of excised human skin to assess the bioequivalence of topical products. Skin Pharmacol Physiol 2009;22(5):276–86.

17. Lehman PA, Raney SG, Franz TJ. Percutaneous absorption in man: in vitro-in vivo correlation. Skin Pharmacol Physiol 2011;24(4):224–30.

18. Radermacher J, Jentsch D, Scholl MA, et al. Diclofenac concentrations in synovial fluid and plasma after cutaneous application in inflammatory and degenerative joint disease. Br J Clin Pharmacol 1991;31(5):537–41.

19. Search for FDA guidance documents. U.S. Food and Drug Administration. Available at: https://www.fda.gov/regulatory-information/search-fda-guidance-documents. Accessed August 26, 2021.

20. Raney SG, Luke MC. A new paradigm for topical generic drug products: impact on therapeutic access. J Am Acad Dermatol 2020;82(6):1570–1.

Dermatology Drugs for Children—U.S. Food and Drug Administration Perspective

Roselyn E. Epps, MD

KEYWORDS

- Pediatric drug development • Best Pharmaceuticals for Children Act (BPCA)
- Pediatric Research Equity Act (PREA)

KEY POINTS

- Drug regulations have increased clinical trials and labeling for the pediatric population.
- Clinical trials in pediatric drug development remain limited.
- More research is needed to address the delays in clinical trials and deficits in labeling information in the pediatric population.

INTRODUCTION

Children have always been treated for symptoms, illnesses, and diseases at home and in the health care setting. Although early drug development evolved due to necessity after serious or lethal events involving children, the pediatric population was not included in legislation crafted in response to these events. Regulations did not address the drug development regulation needs of the pediatric population specifically until later in the twentieth century. In this article, an overview of significant historical regulations affecting drug development in children, US Food and Drug Administration (FDA) regulatory authorities responsible for pediatric dermatology drugs, and recent trends in pediatric dermatology drug development are discussed.

EARLY REGULATORY HISTORY: A "FREE-FOR-ALL"

Everyone wishes to calm a crying baby. Mrs Winslow's Soothing Syrup was marketed for teething and colicky babies in 1849. The company claimed that this product would greatly facilitate the process of teething, alleviate pain and spasmodic action, regulate the bowels, and "give rest to mothers and relief and health to infants." At that time, there was no requirement to list ingredients or test for efficacy or safety. Unfortunately, Mrs Winslow's Soothing Syrup contained morphine and alcohol, resulting in coma, addiction, and death in infants.[1]

Following the deaths of children from biological products related to diphtheria antitoxin and tetanus in St. Louis, MO and Camden, New Jersey, the Biologics Control Act of 1902 enacted premarket licensing authority under the predecessor of the National Institutes of Health (NIH) for therapeutic agents of biological origin. The Biologics Control Act mandated annual licensing of establishments to manufacture and sell vaccines, sera, and antitoxins in interstate commerce.

Drug regulatory functions began in earnest with the passage of the 1906 Pure Food and Drugs Act. This law defined drugs in accordance with the standards of strength, quality, and purity in the United States Pharmacopoeia and the National Formulary, and were not to be sold in any other condition unless the specific variations from the

U.S. Food and Drug Administration, Center for Drug Evaluation and Research, Division of Dermatology and Dentistry, 10903 New Hampshire Avenue, Silver Spring, MD 20903, USA
E-mail address: Roselyn.Epps@fda.hhs.gov

Dermatol Clin 40 (2022) 289–296
https://doi.org/10.1016/j.det.2022.02.004
0733-8635/22/Published by Elsevier Inc.

applicable standards were plainly stated on the label. Although the law prohibited interstate commerce in adulterated and misbranded food and drugs, it did not prohibit the sale of drugs that were not tested for safety and efficacy. The law was enforced by the Bureau of Chemistry in the Department of Agriculture; the Bureau became the United States Food, Drug and Insecticide Administration in 1927, which was designated as the US FDA in 1930.

The Federal Food, Drug, and Cosmetic Act (FDCA) of 1938 was passed after the deaths of 107 patients, many of them children, due to Elixir Sulfanilamide in 1937. Untested diethylene glycol, chemically related to antifreeze, was used to dissolve sulfanilamide into a liquid formulation and for good flavor and resulted in poisoning and deaths after ingestion. The FDCA required proof that any new drug was *safe* before it could be marketed and included a New Drugs section, which is the foundation for drug regulation today.[2]

Thalidomide, marketed as a sleeping pill, was associated with reports of congenital malformations in thousands of babies born in Europe. In 1962, FDA medical officer Frances O. Kelsey, M.D., Ph.D., prevented the marketing of the teratogenic drug thalidomide in the United States. This contributed to Congress passing the Kefauver-Harris Drug Amendments to the FDCA in 1962. The Kefauver-Harris amendments stated that before marketing a drug, applicants need to provide substantial evidence not only of safety but also of *effectiveness* from adequate and well-controlled studies for the product's intended use. In addition, FDCA amendments stated that drugs not tested in children should not be used in children.

THE ORPHAN DRUG ACT

In 1983, the Orphan Drug Act (ODA) allowed FDA encouragement of drug research and development for the treatment of *rare diseases*. Patient advocacy groups influenced enacting this law to stimulate industry interest in developing so-called orphan drugs, which have limited financial potential due to the numerically small population to be treated (ie, affects <200,000 persons in United States). The ODA created financial incentives, including tax credits for the costs of clinical research, and 7 years of marketing exclusivity for the first sponsor of a designated orphan product receiving FDA approval for a particular indication and exemption from application fees for FDA drug marketing.[3] Many dermatologic conditions and genodermatoses fall into the rare disease category, and some have received rare disease designation, such as hereditary angioedema,

mastocytosis, hidradenitis suppurativa, and erythropoietic porphyria.[4] The FDA standard for drug approval to treat orphan conditions is the same as more common diseases, which is, substantial evidence of clinical benefit/effectiveness, safety, and product quality will need to be demonstrated.

PEDIATRIC RULES

In 1992, FDA introduced the Pediatric Labeling Rule and proposed extrapolation of efficacy from other data to the pediatric population.

FDA's Pediatric Rule of 1994 was issued to encourage voluntary development of pediatric data. The Pediatric Rule allowed the labeling of drugs for pediatric use based on the following:

- Extrapolation of efficacy in adults to the pediatric population
- Additional pharmacokinetics (PK), pharmacodynamics, and safety studies in pediatric patients, if the course of the disease and the response to the drug in children are similar to that in adults

The Food and Drug Administration Modernization Act (FDAMA) of 1997 amended the Federal Food, Drug, and Cosmetic Act relating to the regulation of drugs as well as food, devices, and biological products.[5] FDAMA created *pediatric exclusivity*, a provision that provides 6-month marketing exclusivity incentive if studies are completed voluntarily in the pediatric population. The Pediatric Rule as proposed by the Agency in 1997 became *mandatory* in 1998; drug and biological products were required to include pediatric assessments if the drug is likely to be used in a "substantial number of pediatric patients" (i.e., 50,000 children) or if it may provide a "meaningful therapeutic benefit." In 2002 due to litigation, a Washington, D.C. Federal Court declared the Pediatric Rule invalid; it was decided that the rule exceeded FDA's statutory authority.[6]

INTERNATIONAL CONSENSUS

In 2000, what is now the International Conference for Harmonisation (ICH) finalized international guidelines addressing the conduct of clinical trials in pediatric populations. The guidelines facilitate the safe and effective use of medicinal products in pediatric patients. Based on the general principles of ICH E−11, FDA adopted this guideline, including the following:

- Pediatric patients should be given drug products that have been properly evaluated for use in the pediatric population.

- Product development programs should include pediatric studies when appropriate.
- Pediatric product development should not delay adult studies or the availability of drugs for adult patients.[7,8]

THE CARROT

In 2002, the BPCA became law. The BPCA is enacted by the Eunice Kennedy Shriver National Institute of Child Health and Human Development, and the overarching goals are as follows:

- To encourage the pharmaceutical industry to perform pediatric studies to support drug and biological programs, and to improve labeling for patented drug products used in children, by granting an additional 6 months patent exclusivity.
- For NIH to prioritize therapeutic areas and sponsor clinical trials and other research for off-patent drug products that need further study in children.[9]

BPCA (505A) studies are *voluntary*. Section 505A of the FDCA allows identification of off-patent drugs needing further study in children and funds research to fill gaps in knowledge regarding pediatric therapeutics. Data derived from BPCA studies must be included in labeling. FDA encourages completing the studies in children, resulting in additional 6-month marketing exclusivity on successful completion, which is financially beneficial for the sponsor.

THE STICK

In 2003, Pediatric Research Equity Act (PREA) became law. In contrast to BPCA, PREA (505B) studies are *required* and apply to drugs for approved indications only. Pediatric studies conducted under PREA must be labeled; PREA reestablished many components of the FDA's 1998 pediatric rule. Orphan products became exempt from the requirement for pediatric studies (amended in 2017 by the RACE for Children Act), except molecular targets relevant to pediatric cancers.

CONTINUED EVOLUTION OF REGULATIONS—MORE CARROTS

In 2007, the Food and Drug Administration Amendments Act (FDAAA) was signed, expanding the Agency's authority. FDAAA established the Pediatric Review Committee (PeRC), which is mandated by law to internally review all submitted Pediatric Study Plans and Written Requests. When the FDA issues a Written Request, the Agency requests that the sponsor conducts pediatric studies for a product expected to be used in the pediatric population; exclusivity may result. As a result, both negative and positive results of pediatric studies are included in labeling. In addition, BPCA and PREA were reauthorized under FDAAA.

PERMANENT REGULATIONS

BPCA and PREA were reauthorized as *permanent* parts of the Food Drug and Cosmetic Act under the FDA Safety and Innovation Act (FDASIA) in 2012 and under the FDA Reauthorization Act (FDARA) in 2017. Together, BPCA and PREA continue to coordinate the procurement of adequate pediatric efficacy and safety data for labeling. The Pediatric Advisory Committee (PAC) was *permanently* reauthorized under FDASIA.

THE FOOD AND DRUG ADMINISTRATION TODAY

FDA's mission includes protecting the public health by ensuring the safety, efficacy, and security of human and veterinary drugs, biological products, and medical devices. FDA is within the Department of Health and Human Services, part of the Executive Branch of US Government. The laws of the United States, passed by Congress, are organized by subject into the United States Code; the Federal Food, Drug, and Cosmetic Act and subsequent amending statutes are codified in Title 21 of the Code of Federal Regulations. As a regulatory Agency, FDA must respond to regulations from the legislative branch.

FDA divisions, committees, and authorities work together to evaluate and regulate dermatologic drugs and their use in the pediatric population. Prominent "team" members are described later.

The Division of Dermatology and Dentistry (DDD) resides within the Office of New Drugs. As a review division in the Center for Drug Evaluation and Research, DDD regulates Investigational New Drug Applications, New Drug Applications, and Biologics Licensing Applications for drugs and biologics intended for the prevention and treatment of dermatologic and dental conditions. DDD reviews conditions relevant to the pediatric population, including those listed in **Table 1**.

ESTABLISHING EFFECTIVENESS

"Substantial evidence" has been defined in the Food, Drug, and Cosmetic Act as "evidence consisting of adequate and well-controlled (A&WC) investigations… on the basis of which it could fairly and responsibly be concluded by such experts that the drug will have the effect it purports or is

Table 1
Leading conditions seen in the pediatric population reviewed in the Division of Dermatology and Dentistry

Acne	Immunobullous Diseases
Atopic dermatitis	Infestations/head Lice
Condyloma acuminata	Mucositis
Dental caries	Psoriasis
Gingivitis	Verruca vulgaris
Hidradenitis suppurativa	Wound healing/ulcers

Adapted from http://inside.fda.gov:9003/CDER/OfficeofNewDrugs/ONDClinical/OfficeofImmunologyandInflammation OII/ucm64 4916.htm; *with permission.*

represented to have under the conditions of use…". This has generally been interpreted as evidence from at least 2 A&WC trials; however, the regulations allow for flexibility and scientific judgment in applying the standard and in determining the kind and type of data required to be provided for a particular drug to meet the statutory standards.[10]

Unfortunately, the untested pediatric population became a cohort described as "therapeutic orphans," not enrolled in clinical trials and without data to support therapeutic dosing and regimens.[11] As a result, general off-label drug use has continued in children, as marketed drugs were used regardless of data availability.

MODELING AND EXTRAPOLATION

Under the Pediatric Exclusivity Provision passed in 1997, FDA sometimes extrapolates efficacy findings from adults to the pediatric population when designing pediatric drug-development programs. Extrapolation has resulted in additional data for labeling to benefit the pediatric population. The Agency reviewed 370 pediatric studies submitted to the FDA between 1998 and 2008. In response to Written Requests for 166 products, extrapolation of efficacy from adult data occurred for 137 (82.5%) of the drug products. In addition, 84 (61%) of the drug products obtained a new pediatric indication or extension into a new age group. For the 29 products where there was no extrapolation, only 10 (34%) obtained a new pediatric labeling. For example, in dermatology extrapolation by model-informed drug development for adalimumab treatment of hidradenitis suppurativa in adolescents has shown success; this method can be pursued for other conditions on a case-by-case basis.

Exposure–response (E–R) modeling leverages adult data to support pediatric trial design and drug approval. Multiple E-R studies for pediatric populations were submitted to FDA between 2007 and 2018. The focus of applications of E–R evaluation in pediatric drug development programs is as follows:

- supporting pediatric extrapolation when the E–R relationships are similar between the pediatric and adult populations;
- dose selection to balance the risk–benefit profile based on the change in efficacy and safety response with different exposure levels
- approval of a new formulation, new dosing regimen, or new route of administration

Dermatology indications that applied E-R modeling for dose selection in the pediatric population include terbinafine for tinea capitis and omalizumab for chronic idiopathic urticaria.

PHARMACOKINETIC CONSIDERATIONS

Although children are not small adults, there can be physiologic comparability for some products in the pediatric population. Pharmacokinetic testing supports use and dosing in drug development. Confirmatory pharmacokinetic data may be obtained through sampling during pivotal efficacy and safety trials. Under FDAAA 2007, a review of 126 products with at least 1 pediatric trial completed identified 92 products with adolescent indications concordant with adult indications. Of these 92 products, 87 (94.5%) have identical adolescent and adult dosing. In some instances, adolescent doses were derived from adult data without the need for a dedicated pharmacokinetic study. Yet because of the complexities of drug development, some products may require a more extensive pharmacokinetic evaluation in the adolescent population. The approach to PK should be determined on a case-by-case basis.

In addition to DDD, there are other FDA offices with regulatory authority pertinent to dermatologic products used in the pediatric population.

- The Office of Orphan Product Development (OOPD) implements components of the ODA. The OOPD mission is to advance the evaluation and development of products (drugs, biologics, devices, or medical foods) that demonstrate promise for the diagnosis and/or treatment of rare diseases or conditions. OOPD provides incentives for sponsors to develop products for rare diseases through orphan drug designation and orphan drug exclusivity. The program has successfully enabled the development and marketing of drugs for pediatric dermatologic diseases and conditions. In addition, the Orphan Product Grant Program awards research grants to support product development clinical trials and for disease natural history studies.
- The Office of Infectious Diseases reviews many topical and systemic antiinfective drugs used in pediatric and general dermatology (eg, mupirocin).
- Office of Nonprescription Drugs reviews over-the-counter (OTC) products and oversees the development, review, and regulation of nonprescription products (marketed under OTC monographs and under NDAs). This broad oversight portfolio includes numerous products such as dandruff shampoos, antiitch products, certain acne and wart medications, and sunscreens.
- Office of Generic Drugs ensures high-quality, affordable generic drugs are available to the American public. FDA-approved generic drugs account for about 90% of prescriptions filled in the United States for all populations.
- The Office of Surveillance and Epidemiology monitors and evaluates the safety profiles of drugs available to the US population throughout the drug product life cycle. The Division of Pharmacovigilance uses a variety of surveillance tools to detect safety signals and assess safety-related issues for all marketed drug and therapeutic biological products. The Division of Epidemiology conducts active drug safety surveillance and epidemiologic studies using observational data resources and reviews drug safety–related epidemiologic study protocols and study reports that are required of manufacturers as postmarketing requirements and commitments.

The Pediatric Review Committee (PeRC), established under FDAAA, is within the Division of Pediatrics and Maternal Health. PeRC is mandated to carry out activities related to BPCA and PREA. The committee consists of FDA employees with expertise in pediatrics, biopharmacology, statistics, chemistry, legal issues, pediatric ethics, and other appropriate expertise.[12]

The Office of Pediatric Therapeutics (OPT), located in the Commissioner's Office, is responsible for the coordination and facilitation of all activities of the FDA that may have any effect on a pediatric population or may in any other way involve pediatric issues. OPT focuses on 4 areas pertaining to pediatrics: scientific, ethical, safety, and international. In addition, OPT manages the PAC activities.

The PAC advises and makes recommendations to the Commissioner of Food and Drugs regarding pediatric research conducted under sections 351, 409I, and 499 of the Public Health Service Act and sections 501, 502, 505, 505A, and 505B of the Federal Food, Drug, and Cosmetic Act. PAC advises and makes recommendations as they relate to pediatric therapeutics (including drugs and biological products) and medical devices, pediatric research, pediatric ethical issues, and other matters involving pediatrics for which the FDA has regulatory responsibility. The Committee also advises and makes recommendations to the Secretary.

PUBLIC–PRIVATE PARTNERSHIP

The FDA entered public–private partnerships with the nonprofit Critical Path Institute and other stakeholders, including the European Medicine Agency, in 2005. The purpose of the collaboration is to promote and foster medical product innovation through the exchange of scientific information and collaboration in research and education. Multiple area-specific programs seek to accelerate medical product development through the creation of new standards of data, measurement, and methods to aid in the scientific evaluation of efficacy and safety of new therapies.[13]

BENEFITS FROM LEGISLATION

BPCA and PREA legislation have resulted in increased drug development and drug product studies in the pediatric population (**Table 2**). Annually, BPCA meets and prioritizes drugs for study and funding and accepts public recommendations for studies. Specific therapeutics are selected for study after discussion and review. Under BPCA, working groups by specialty have made recommendations, including the Dermatology Therapeutics Working Group. After the study ends, FDA reviews completed studies for inclusion in labeling (**Table 3**). BPCA-related labeling changes relevant to dermatologic indications are listed in **Table 4**.

Table 2
Total pediatric studies conducted under BPCA and PREA: 2012 to present

Program	Total Number of Products Studied
BPCA	58
PREA	312
BPCA and PREA	9

Data from https://www.fda.gov/drugs/development-resources/reviews-pediatric-studies-conducted-under-bpca-and-prea-2012-present Current as of April 12, 2021.

The DDD has issued 26 Written Requests for marketing exclusivity.[14] Pediatric studies conducted in response to Written Request issued under BPCA with Pediatric assessments conducted under PREA are listed in **Box 1**.

DISCUSSION

For many decades, parents and children, prescribers, pharmacists, professional and advocacy groups, and regulatory authorities have promoted and advocated for safe use of therapeutics in the pediatric population. Although progress has been made, there is still an unmet need for safe, developmentally appropriate drug development and increased labeling for the pediatric population. Clinical trials in pediatrics still remain limited. Pediatric drug development presents many challenges, including small populations to study, developmental and maturational changes, phenotypic variability, poorly understood natural history, lack of appropriate biomarkers, outcome measures and endpoints, and difficulties in identifying appropriate control groups.[15] After drug approval in adults, there is an average delay of 9 years until drug approval for pediatric labeling.[16]

Because of the lack of data, many drugs prescribed for the pediatric population and pediatric dermatology indications have been prescribed off-label. It has been stated that greater than 50% of drugs approved lack pediatric labeling information.[17] Data analysis from the National Ambulatory Medical Care Surveys from 2001 to

Table 3
Drugs reviewed under BPCA and PREA relevant to dermatology indications: 2012 to present

Acyclovir 5%, Hydrocortisone 1%—Xerese	Etanercept-szzs—Erelzi
Acyclovir sodium—Zovirax	Fluticasone propionate Lotion—Cutivate
Adalimumab—Humira	Glycopyrronium—Qbrexza
Adalimumab-fkjp—Hulio—plaque psoriasis	Halobetasol—Propionate Ultravate
Adalimumab-atto—Amjevita	Infliximab-axxq—Avsola
Adapalene and benzoyl peroxide—Epiduo	Infliximab-dyyb—Inflectra
Adapalene and benzoyl peroxide—Epiduo Forte	Infliximab-abda—Renflexis
Belimumab—Benlysta (SLE)	Ipilimumab—Yervoy
Calcipotriene—SORILUX Foam	Ixekizumab—Taltz
Calcipotriene—SORILUX	Minocycline—Amzeeq
Calcipotriene and Betamethasone dipropionate—Taclonex ointment	Naftifine hydrochloride—Naftin Cream
Calcipotriene and Betamethasone dipropionate—Taclonex topical suspension	Sarecycline—Seysara
Calcipotriene and betamethasone—Enstilar	Spinosad—Natroba
Calcitriol—Vectical	Tacrolimus—Astagraf XL
Crisaborole Ointment, 2%—Eucrisa	Tavaborole—Kerydin
Dapsone—Aczone	Tazarotene—Arazlo
Daptomycin—Cubicin	Tedizolid phosphate—Sivextro
Doxycycline hyclate delayed-release—Doryx	Tretinoin lotion—Altreno
Dupilumab—Dupixent	Trifarotene—Akli
Econazole nitrate—Ecoz	Ustekinumab—Stelara
Etanercept—Enbrel	—

Data from https://www.fda.gov/drugs/development-resources/reviews-pediatric-studies-conducted-under-bpca-and-prea-2012-present Current as of April 12, 2021.

Table 4
BCPA studies completed/NIH funded with pediatric labeling changes relevant to dermatologic therapy

Drug	Change
Acyclovir	Update Dosage and Administration, Clinical Pharmacology, and Adverse Reactions sections of the label
Bactrim	Add pediatric pharmacokinetic data to the Clinical Pharmacology section
Clindamycin	Add clinical pharmacology and dosage information for obese children (clindamycin should be dosed based on total body weight)
Doxycycline	Add pediatric data to Pharmacokinetics subsection of Clinical Pharmacology section

Data from https://www.fda.gov/drugs/development-resources/nih-funded-pediatric-labeling-changes-drugs-studied-under-409i-process Current as of September 28, 2020.

Box 1
Dermatology products studied in response to Written Request, 2012 to present

Adapalene and benzoyl peroxide—Epiduo

Adapalene and benzoyl peroxide—Epiduo Forte

Crisaborole Ointment, 2%—Eucrisa

Dapsone—Aczone

Econazole nitrate—Ecoza

Fluticasone propionate Lotion—Cutivate

Glycopyrronium—Qbrexza

Ixekizumab—Taltz

Luliconazole—Luzu

Naftifine hydrochloride—Naftin

Ozenoxacin—Xepi

Sarecycline—Seysara

Tavaborole—Kerydin

Tazarotene—Aralzo

Tretinoin lotion—Altreno

Ustekinumab—Stelara

Adapted from https://www.fda.gov/drugs/development-resources/reviews-pediatric-studies-conducted-under-bpca-and-prea-2012-present. Accessed April 9, 2021; with permission.

2004 outpatient visits for children from birth to 17 years revealed that 62% of outpatient pediatric visits included off-label prescribing, and 67% of dermatologic medication prescriptions were off-label.[18]

The promotion of research has attempted to address some of the deficits and delays regarding pediatric drug development and therapeutics. Since BPCA and PREA were enacted, dermatology drug development programs are prominent in evaluation and labeling for the pediatric population. Acne, atopic dermatitis, and psoriasis are a few conditions in which drug development programs routinely address and embrace product efficacy and safety in the pediatric population. The Office of Orphan Drug Products has facilitated drug development in rare diseases through designation programs and grants to facilitate drug development in rare diseases.

For future drug development and to support efficacy, additional research including the pathophysiology and pharmacokinetics of drug products in the pediatric population is critical. A drug development program must take into account percutaneous and systemic absorption, as well as clearance and the physiologic development of the renal and hepatic systems. In addition to older children, more data are needed to support safe and effective use of drugs in neonates and infants. To obtain data, an understanding of and strategies for considering pathophysiology, drug disposition, biomarkers, and clinically meaningful endpoints is critical.

In addition, strategies for using data in adults such as extrapolation and modeling can support product use in the pediatric population; additional study and review are needed to advance and strengthen these methods.

Laws and regulations regarding pediatric drug development continue to change and evolve, as amendments and additional legislation are passed. Although BPCA and PREA implementation have increased the number of pediatric studies and data, there are delays in clinical trials and deficits in labeling information. Through drug labeling for pediatric populations, prescribers, patients, and other stakeholders can make informed recommendations and decisions regarding treatments to benefit children.

DISCLOSURE

The author has nothing to disclose.

CLINICS CARE POINTS

- There is an unmet need for safe, developmentally appropriate dermatology drug development and labeling for the pediatric population.
- Many drugs used for the pediatric popoulation and pediatric dermatology indications have been prescribed off-label.
- Additional research is needed, including the pathophysiology and pharmacokinetics of dermatology drug products in the pediatric population.

REFERENCES

1. Available at: https://www.accessdata.fda.gov/scripts/cderworld/index.cfm?action=newdrugs:main&unit=4&lesson=1&topic=3
2. Ballentine, C. Sulfanilamide Disaster. FDA Consumer magazine, June 1981, https://www.fda.gov/about-fda/histories-product-regulation/sulfanilamide-disaster.
3. 21 CFR 316.20.
4. Available at: https://www.fda.gov/industry/developing-products-rare-diseases-conditions
5. Pub.L. 105-115.
6. Available at: https://www.govinfo.gov/content/pkg/USCOURTS-dcd-1_00-cv-02898/pdf/USCOURTS-dcd-1_00-cv-02898-0.pdf
7. Available at: http://www.fda.gov/Drugs/GuidanceComplianceRegulatoryInformation/Guidances/ucm065005.htm
8. Available at: https://www.fda.gov/regulatory-information/search-fda-guidance-documents/e11-clinical-investigation-medicinal-products-pediatric-population
9. Best Pharmaceuticals for Children Act (BPCA). Available at: https://www.nichd.nih.gov/research/supported/bpca. Accessed April 9, 2021.
10. Guidance for Industry "Providing Clinical Evidence of Effectiveness for Human Drug and Biological Products". Available at: https://www.fda.gov/regulatory-information/search-fda-guidance-documents/providing-clinical-evidence-effectiveness-human-drug-and-biological-products.
11. Shirkey H. Therapeutic orphans. Pediatr 1999;104(3 Pt 2):583–4.
12. PeRC Information Page. Available at: http://inside.fda.gov:9003/CDER/OfficeofNewDrugs/ONDClinical/OfficeofRareDiseasesPediatricsUrologyandReproductiveMedicineORPURM/DivisionofPediatricsandMaternalHealthDPMH/ucm027829.htm. Assessed April 9, 2021.
13. Available at: https://c-path.org/. Assessed April 22, 2021.
14. US FDA Pediatric Exclusivity Statistics. Available at: https://www.fda.gov/drugs/development-resources/pediatric-exclusivity-statistics. Accessed April 9, 2021.
15. Mulugeta LY, Yao L, Mould D, et al. Leveraging Big Data in Pediatric Development Programs: Proceedings From the 2016 American College of Clinical Pharmacology Annual Meeting Symposium. Clin Pharmacol Ther 2018;104(1):81–7.
16. Tanaudommongkon I, John Miyagi S, Green DJ, et al. Combined Pediatric and Adult Trials Submitted to the US Food and Drug Administration 2012-2018. Clin Pharmacol Ther 2020;108(5):1018–25.
17. Hudgins JD, Bacho MA, Olsen KL, et al. Pediatric drug information available at the time of new drug approvals: A cross-sectional analysis. Pharmacoepidemiol Drug Saf 2018;27(2):161–7.
18. Bazzano AT, Mangione-Smith R, Schonlau M, et al. Off-label prescribing to children in the United States outpatient setting. Acad Pediatr 2009;9(2):81–8.

Regulation of Medical Devices for Dermatology

Shlomit Halachmi, MD, PhD[a],*, Laura Marquart, MD[b]

KEYWORDS

- Medical device • Laser • Energy-based device • Light-based device • Dermal filler
- Soft tissue filler • Wound care product • Chronic wound

KEY POINTS

- A medical device is defined by its intended use/indications for use and by its means of action.
- Most devices in dermatology practice are moderate- to high-risk Class II devices, including electro-surgical and light-based devices, sutures, and certain diagnostic aids.
- Class II devices are cleared for marketing when they are determined to be substantially equivalent to a legally marketed predicate device.
- High-risk, Class III medical devices in dermatology require extensive premarket and postmarket assessment and annual reports to ensure safety and effectiveness.

INTRODUCTION

Dermatologic care is replete with device-based procedures, from those that assist in diagnosis (eg, dermoscopes, Woods light, and skin lesion analyzers) to a broad range of therapeutic modalities (eg, light and non-light energy-based devices, wound care products, and dermal fillers).[1] In the United States, all medical devices are regulated by the Food and Drug Administration (FDA), but different devices are subject to different regulations. This article reviews the history of medical device regulation, explains how medical devices are defined and classified, and outlines the regulatory pathways of current dermatologic devices.

HISTORY

Federal regulation of food and drugs began when the Pure Food and Drugs Act in 1906 was implemented to regulate interstate commerce of food and drugs that are misbranded (having false or misleading labeling) or adulterated (bearing a deleterious substance). Oversight was expanded in 1938 through the Federal Food, Drug, and Cosmetic Act (FD&C Act) to include cosmetics and therapeutic medical devices and in 1968 to include radiation-emitting products. However, medical devices presented a different set of regulatory issues than drugs. Therefore, significant definitions and regulations for medical devices were enacted in 1976 with the passing of the Medical Device Amendments to the FD&C Act.

These amendments provide the basis for how medical devices are regulated today. They outline, among other aspects:

- Risk-based stratification of medical devices, as Class I, II, or III
- Regulatory pathways for new medical devices, generally requiring premarket review of new Class II and Class III medical devices
- Assessment of both safety and effectiveness of medical devices
  - With respect to the patients and providers for whose use the device is intended;
  - With respect to the conditions of use (e.g. setting, disease) prescribed; and

a Center for Devices and Radiological Health, US Food and Drug Administration, White Oak Building 66, Room 4529, 10903 New Hampshire Avenue, Silver Spring, MD 20993, USA; b Center for Devices and Radiological Health, US Food and Drug Administration, White Oak Building 66, Room 4556, 10903 New Hampshire Avenue, Silver Spring, MD 20993, USA
* Corresponding author.
E-mail address: shlomit.halachmi@fda.hhs.gov

Dermatol Clin 40 (2022) 297–305
https://doi.org/10.1016/j.det.2022.02.005
0733-8635/22/Published by Elsevier Inc.

○ Weighing probable benefit from the use of the device to health against probable risk of injury from the use of the device

After the Amendments were enacted, FDA began categorizing all previously existing medical devices and classifying each device type by risk into Class I, II, or III. Not all preamendments devices (ie, devices legally marketed before the enactment of the Medical Device Amendments of 1976) have been classified. Conversely, new technologies and medical uses for devices have developed since 1976. These are classified before marketing.

There have been numerous subsequent amendments to the FD&C Act, including notably the Safe Medical Devices Act of 1990, FDA Modernization Act of 1997, Medical Device User Fee and Modernization Act of 2002, FDA Amendments Act of 2007, FDA Safety and Innovation Act of 2012, the 21st Century Cures Act of 2016, and FDA Reauthorization Act of 2017.

DEFINITIONS
Medical Device

Section 201(h) of the FD&C Act defines the term "device" as an instrument, apparatus, implement, machine, contrivance, implant, in vitro reagent, or other similar or related article, including a component part, or accessory, which is

(1) Recognized in the official National Formulary, or the United States Pharmacopoeia, or any supplement to them
(2) Intended for use in the diagnosis of disease or other conditions, or in the cure, mitigation, treatment, or prevention of disease, in man or other animals
(3) Intended to affect the structure or any function of the body of man or other animals
  • Which does not achieve its primary intended purposes through chemical action within or on the body of man or other animals
  • Which is not dependent on being metabolized for the achievement of its primary intended purposes. The term "device" does not include software functions excluded pursuant to section 520(o).

Note that medical devices may be part of a combination product, such as a product that is a combination of a device and drug or device and biologic.[2] Combination products include single-entity products (prefilled drug delivery systems or drug-eluting devices), copackaged products (separate drug and device within same package), or cross-labeled products (drug for use in photodynamic therapy).[3] Combination products are outside the scope of this article.

Intended Use

Intended Use describes the general purpose of a device as a "tool" (eg, for coagulation of soft tissues), as intended by the device manufacturer.[4] The Intended Use of a device can affect how the device is regulated and may be determined based on device labeling claims, advertising materials, or other statements made by the manufacturer.

Indication for Use

The Indication for Use (IFU) is a description of the disease or condition the device will diagnose, treat, prevent, cure, or mitigate. The IFU may include a description of the patient population for which the device is intended.[5]

For example, the IFU of a device may be "to promote hair growth in females with androgenetic alopecia who have Ludwig-Savin Classifications I-II and Fitzpatrick Skin Phototypes I-IV." If a device has multiple components, for example, different wavelengths or handpieces, each may be cleared with its own IFU, for example, "The Q-switched 1064 nm wavelength is indicated for removal of black and blue tattoo inks; the long-pulse 532 nm wavelength is indicated for treatment of vascular lesions."

Class I, II, III, and De Novo

The FD&C Act established 3 categories of medical devices (Class I, Class II, and Class III) and requires FDA to classify devices intended for human use into one of these categories.[6] The tiered classification is based on risk and includes associated level of regulatory control necessary to mitigate that risk.

Class I A device is Class I if general controls (a set of requirements for all medical devices) are sufficient to provide reasonable assurance of the safety and effectiveness of the device. Class I devices are generally considered to be low- to moderate-risk devices (ie, not life-supporting or life-sustaining, not of substantial importance in preventing impairment of health, and does not present potential unreasonable risk of illness of injury).

Most Class I devices are exempt from FDA premarket review. In dermatology, these include medical examination tables, microscopes, skin markers, shoe covers, manual surgical instruments for general use, cannulas for general and plastic surgery, percutaneous biopsy devices, some wound dressings, silicone sheeting, and needle-type epilators.[7]

Class II Class II devices are generally moderate- to high-risk devices for which general controls alone are insufficient to provide reasonable assurance of safety and effectiveness and for which there is sufficient information to establish special controls to provide such assurance. The special controls may include performance standards, postmarket surveillance, or patient registries and may be described in FDA regulations or guidance documents.

Class II devices are generally subject to premarket notification (PMN) or 510(k), named for section 510(k) of the FD&C Act.[8] The term "premarket notification" is used because this section of the FD&C Act called for manufacturers to submit a notification of intent to FDA at least 90 days before bringing a Class II device into interstate commerce.

A device subject to PMN is cleared to be marketed when the manufacturer demonstrates that the device is *substantially equivalent* (SE) in safety and effectiveness to a predicate device. A predicate device may be a device that was legally marketed before May 28, 1976 (the date of enactment of the Medical Device Amendments of 1976), generally referred to as preamendments devices, or a more recently cleared Class II device (**Fig. 1**). Currently, legally marketed Class II devices are often cleared based on a predicate device that was in turn based on a predicate device that traces its evolution from a device that was legally marketed before May 28, 1976.

By way of example, modern lasers used in dermatology are derived, regulatorily, from a chain of SE predicate devices that originated from a small number of preamendments devices, including argon and carbon dioxide lasers.[9]

In addition to lasers, examples of Class II devices in dermatology include other energy-based devices, digital dermoscopes and other aids to visualization, sutures, and devices applied for wound management. A limited list of Class II devices are exempted from PMN, such as surgical lamps and drapes.[7] Not all ancillary items for procedures are exempt, however. For example, surgical masks, defined by claims of filtration as well as fluid resistance, are medical devices subject to 510(k) review.

Class III Class III devices, reviewed under premarket approval (PMA), are associated with the highest potential risk. A device is designated Class III if general and special controls do not provide sufficient assurance of safety and effectiveness, and if, in addition, the device is life-supporting or life-sustaining, or of substantial importance in preventing impairment of health, or presents a potential unreasonable risk of illness or injury. The PMA process involves greater premarket oversight of device design, manufacturing, and clinical performance.

PMA-approved devices are subject to additional postmarket requirements, including, but not limited to, submission of annual reports by the device manufacturer. These annual reports may include the number of devices sold (to allow for assessing rate of adverse events reported); reports of published or unpublished data that have come to light; and any changes in labeling or manufacturing. Some PMA-approved devices require additional confirmation of clinical performance in postapproval studies.

Dermal fillers, being implants (devices placed into the body and intended to remain implanted for a period of 30 days or more), and being highly dependent on the manufacturing process, are high risk and regulated as Class III devices, as are certain diagnostic devices and complex wound care products.

De novo De novo classification is an alternate pathway to classify novel medical devices that are determined to be not SE to an existing Class I or II device, or for which there is no legally marketed device to base a determination of substantial equivalence. If the device does not have risks that would place it in Class III, and if risks can be mitigated with special controls, then a De Novo

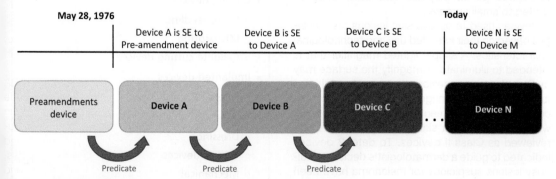

Fig. 1. Schematic of substantial equivalence in 510(k) review. (*Courtesy of* S Halachmi, MD, PhD, and L Marquart, MD of FDA, Silver Spring, MD).

may be appropriate. De Novo requests are reviewed by FDA, and if granted, the new device can be legally marketed and can serve as a predicate device for future 510(k) submissions.

Examples of dermatologic devices that entered the market through the De Novo classification pathway include focused ultrasound for aesthetic use and use of cooling for body contouring. Home use radiofrequency for treatment of wrinkles was also introduced to market initially under a De Novo request because the intended user of the device changed from trained professional to consumer.

Food and Drug Administration–Approved, Cleared, Granted, Authorized, Registered, Listed
These terms have distinct meanings regarding whether and how FDA has reviewed a product:

- "FDA-Approved" denotes that a medical device has been reviewed as a Class III device in a premarket approval submission and received marketing authorization.
- "FDA-Cleared" is the term used to indicate that a Class I or Class II device was FDA-reviewed in a 510(k) premarket notification and received marketing authorization.
- "Granted" indicates a device was reviewed by FDA in a De Novo request and received marketing authorization.
- "Registration and listing" means all medical device manufacturers and certain importers must register their establishment and list their device or devices, regardless of whether they are Class I, II, or III. Therefore, claims that a device is "FDA listed" or that an establishment is "FDA registered" does not denote approval or clearance of the device by FDA.

DEVICES IN DERMATOLOGY
Diagnostic

Many of the common instruments used in dermatology diagnostic procedures are Class I devices, to include punch biopsies and other supplies related to small surgeries.

Devices used to assess skin lesions are classified based on their intended use and technological characteristics. A simple lighted magnifier that is intended to illuminate or magnify the surface may be Class I, whereas devices that provide additional functions, such as image acquisition and/or processing, or enhancement of specific components within an image of a skin lesion, are likely to be reviewed as Class II devices. To date, 2 devices indicated to guide a dermatologist's decision to biopsy lesions suspicious for melanoma have been approved as Class III devices.

Therapeutic

Most therapeutic dermatology devices are reviewed by the Office of Surgical and Infection Control Devices. Discussion of similar technologies that are marketed for physical therapy or gynecologic use, but also applied in dermatology, is outside the scope of this article.

Devices in dermatology can be categorized by their technology and by their Intended Use or Indications for Use. The technologies most commonly applied can be categorized broadly as in **Box 1**.

Box 1
Categories of dermatology medical devices

Energy-based devices:

- Heating
  - Light-based
    - Laser
    - Intense Pulsed Light (IPL)
    - Photobiomodulation (formerly low-level light therapy [LLLT])
  - Electrical:
    - Radiofrequency (RF)
    - Electrosurgical
  - Microwave
  - Ultrasound
- Cooling
  - Cryotherapy
  - Contact cooling
- Vibration/pressure
  - Ultrasound
  - Massage
  - Shockwave
- Magnetic Pulse Field

Non-energy-based devices:

- Cutting devices
  - Microneedling
  - Microcoring
  - Cellulite cutting devices
- Implanted devices
  - Fillers
- Wound care devices
  - Dressings
  - Topical devices
  - Mechanical

Energy-based devices

Energy-based devices in dermatology are largely Class II devices. The review assesses whether the information provided for that the proposed device demonstrates substantial equivalence to a predicate device that is already cleared for the same Intended Use and that has similar technological characteristics. FDA reviews device performance for each IFU individually. A device with a single component (e.g., one wavelength or one handpiece) may be cleared for one or more Intended Uses or Indications for Use. For example, a long-pulse alexandrite laser (755nm) may be cleared for permanent hair reduction, treatment of benign vascular lesions, and wrinkles. A device with multiple components (e.g., multiple modes, wavelengths, or handpieces) may have separate clearance(s) for each component. For example, a laser system may be cleared for specific IFUs for each wavelength, such as 532nm wavelength for vascular lesions and 1064nm wavelength for wrinkles.

Device clearance is based on a review of performance, including both safety and effectiveness. Benefit-risk consideration can result in IFUs that are limited to certain Fitzpatrick phototypes, specific body sites, specific gender, or to certain disease subtypes or severity (for example, mild to moderate inflammatory acne). The language cleared is based on the totality of the information available for the known or expected effectiveness and the known or potential safety concerns.

Special Topics in Energy-Based Devices

Accessories

Accessories for energy-based devices are considered medical devices.[10] Such accessory devices may include nanoparticles that absorb laser light within a target space and devices intended to clear an optical path for enhanced light delivery.

Home use devices

The Intended Use of a product includes whether the product is used by a trained provider or by a layperson, as in the case of a home use device. Safety and effectiveness of a device in a home use setting requires consideration for how an untrained user may apply the device. Therefore, FDA may request additional information to support correct use, safety, and effectiveness for devices that may be intended for use at home.

Over the counter

Most dermatology devices reviewed under Class II are cleared for prescription (Rx) use. Providers may prescribe them for use at home, and therefore, some home use devices are Rx devices. However, home use devices may be cleared for over-the-counter (OTC) use. In such cases, assessment of safety and effectiveness of a device requires additional consideration for how potential lay users may use the device. Therefore, for OTC devices, FDA requests additional information to demonstrate that an average consumer can correctly "self-select" (determine whether the product is applicable to their condition, safe for them to use, and likely to provide the desired outcome, can comprehend the instructions, and can use the device correctly.

Sunlamp products

All UV-emitting products intended for human exposure are currently regulated as medical devices. Before 2014, UV-emitting devices intended for treatment of skin disease were regulated as Class II, whereas UV lamps intended to tan the skin were regulated as Class I and exempt from PMN. In 2014, FDA defined the terms "sunlamp products" (devices designed to incorporate UV lamps with wavelengths of 200–400 nm, to induce skin tanning) and "UV lamps intended for use in sunlamp products" (any lamp that produces UV radiation in the wavelength interval of 200–400 nm in air).[11] Furthermore, FDA reclassified UV lamps intended to tan the skin from Class I (general controls) exempt from PMN to Class II (special controls), making them subject to PMN. In the reclassification, FDA designated special controls necessary to provide a reasonable assurance of safety and effectiveness of the device.[12]

Non-energy-based devices

Dermal fillers

Materials Dermal fillers, also known as soft tissue fillers, or wrinkle fillers, are implants intended to remain for at least 30 days and are regulated as Class III (PMA) products.[13] These products may be composed of base materials, which may be absorbable or nonabsorbable (permanent). Others include lidocaine, which is intended to decrease pain related to the injection. A list of FDA-approved fillers as of January 2021 is available in the executive summary the March 23, 2021 Meeting of the General and Plastic Surgery Devices.

FDA has not approved liquid silicone, silicone gel, or polyacrylamide for use as dermal fillers[14] (**Box 2**). In 2017, FDA published a Safety Communication warning against use of injectable silicone owing to reports of its use for body contouring and enhancement, citing risks of infections, scarring, disfigurement, embolism, stroke, and death.[15] Because silicone migrates, adverse events may be distant from the site of injection.

Box 2
Filler materials approved by Food and Drug Administration

Absorbable fillers ("temporary"):

- Collagen: the first dermal fillers approved by FDA, composed of bovine, porcine, or human-based collagen. Before treatment with bovine collagen, each patient first underwent skin testing for hypersensitivity, generally by injection of a small volume of filler into the medial aspect of the forearm.

- Hyaluronic acid (HA): a naturally occurring tissue polysaccharide that swells when combined with water, leading to a filling effect. HA is produced from bacteria or rooster combs and may be cross-linked with 1,4-butanediol diglycidyl ether (BDDE) to increase its stability and longevity, which has been reported to be 6 to 24 months.

- Calcium hydroxylapatite (CaHA): a mineral found in bones and teeth, CaHA lasts approximately 12 months per clinical studies. A carboxymethylcellulose gel carrier suspends the CaHA particles for injection. The gel dissipates in the tissue, leaving the CaHA particles at the injection sites to provide soft tissue augmentation. Because of the presence of calcium, CaHA is visible in radiological imaging. To address the risk of imaging artifacts, FDA requests additional preclinical data as part of the premarket review for CaHA dermal fillers to ensure CaHA does not obscure X-ray findings. CaHA has been approved for use in the face and hands.

- Poly-L-lactic acid (PLLA): a synthetic biodegradable polymer used in absorbable sutures and orthopedic medical devices. PLLA is a long-lasting filler. Its effects become increasingly apparent over time and lasts up to 2 years. It may be injected in a series of treatments over a period of time.

Nonabsorbable fillers ("permanent"):

- Polymethylmethacrylate (PMMA) microspheres: a synthetic biocompatible polymer used in orthopedic, neurosurgical, ophthalmologic, and dental devices. PMMA fillers contain bovine collagen as a carrier of PMMA microspheres and allows even distribution of the microspheres in the target tissue. The collagen is degraded within a few months and replaced by in situ connective tissue between the microspheres. Because of the presence of bovine collagen, some patients may exhibit hypersensitivity. A pretreatment test, by intradermal injection into volar forearm skin, can identify individuals who may be hypersensitive to bovine collagen. Because the microspheres are nonabsorbable, removal is surgical.

Box 3
Approved IFU for Fillers

Absorbable fillers have been approved for

- Correction of nasolabial folds
- Correction of age-related volume deficits in the midface
- Moderate to severe facial wrinkles and folds, such as nasolabial folds and perioral lines
- Augmentation of lips, cheeks, chin
- Volume loss of the dorsal hand
- Correction of contour deficiencies, such as wrinkles and acne scars
- Restoration/correction of the signs of facial fat loss (lipoatrophy) in people with or receiving treatment for human immunodeficiency virus

---

Surgical removal may not be possible and may not rid the body of the silicone.

A list of all approved dermal fillers is available on the PMA Database Search Web site.[16] Dermal fillers for the face can be found under the product code "LMH," and dermal fillers for the hand can be found under product code "PKY." However, some approved fillers may no longer be marketed.

Indications for use of dermal fillers

Dermal fillers are approved for injection into specific body sites, such as the cheeks, chin, lips, hand, and for specific IFUs[17] (**Box 3**).

Nonabsorbable fillers are approved only for nasolabial folds and cheek acne scars.

The FDA recommends against using any injectable filler for body contouring and enhancement procedures, such as,[18]

- Injection into muscle, ligament, or tendon
- Breast augmentation
- Buttock lift or augmentation
- Injections to increase fullness of the feet

FDA provided a review of reported adverse events related to fillers in the March 2021 meeting of the General and Plastic Surgery Devices Panel of the Medical Devices Advisory Committee.[14] Unintentional intravascular injection may lead to tissue necrosis, visual compromise, including blindness, or neurologic sequelae, including stroke.

Note that marketing of dermal fillers for use with blunt-tipped cannulas requires approval for the product to be labeled for use with cannula.

Wound care devices

Wound care devices can be regulated under Class I, Class II, or Class III, or they may be unclassified. Rx wound care products are cleared or approved with specific intended uses, for example, to cover, absorb exudate, create a moist wound environment, or rinse debris. The IFU may state specific wound types, such as pressure ulcers; venous, arterial, or diabetic foot ulcers; or postsurgical wounds. The IFU may also limit use to a severity range, such as first- and second-degree burns, or for a duration.

Rx wound care products may be broadly categorized, within each regulatory Class, as follows.

Class I devices

Simple wound dressings Simple wound dressing products, used to cover a wound, to absorb wound exudate, and/or to control bleeding or fluid loss, to protect against friction, desiccation, or contamination, are Class I, provided they do not contain drugs, biologics, or materials derived from animal sources or exceed limitations of each product's specific regulations as Class I devices.

Devices requiring PMN/510(k)

Wound dressings with drugs These are device-led combination products that were legally marketed in interstate commerce before May 28, 1976 and have not been classified into Class I, II, or III.[19] A discussion of combination products is outside the scope of this article. Briefly, PMN/510(k) is required for these products. Unclassified wound dressings that contain drugs (eg, sodium hypochlorite, silver, polyhexamethylene biguanide) can be categorized into 3 general categories based on the physical state of the dressing:

- Solid wound dressings
- Gels, creams, and ointments
- Liquid wound washes (considered devices because the stream of the liquid provides physical debridement)

Drugs included in these products may have antimicrobial claims. However, the antimicrobial claims are limited to effects within the dressing, for example, to reduce colonization of the dressing or to prolong the shelf life of the dressing.

Skin barrier cream/emulsion Certain skin barrier creams are reviewed as medical devices, rather than drugs, because of their composition and their intended use of "maintaining a moist wound environment." These skin barrier creams may be used to manage various types of dermatoses, including atopic dermatitis, irritant contact dermatitis, and radiation dermatitis.

Class III devices

Interactive wound dressings These products are intended to replace full function of the skin and to promote healing by interaction with the wound. Some may contain biologics or animal-derived components and may be under the oversight of Center for Devices and Radiological Health or FDA's Center for Biologics Evaluation and Research.

Other wound care devices include the following mechanical interventions:

- Compression devices:
  - Compression dressings comprising elastic bandages are Class I exempt.
  - Pneumatic compression devices, intended for reducing wound healing time and of treatment and assistance in healing stasis dermatitis, venous stasis ulcers, or arterial and diabetic leg ulcers, are Class II devices.
- Negative pressure wound therapy devices, including powered or nonpowered devices intended for wound management via application of continual or intermittent negative pressure to the wound for removal of fluids, including wound exudate, irrigation fluids, and infectious materials, are Class II.
  - Low-energy ultrasound wound cleaners use ultrasound energy to vaporize a solution and generate a mist that is used for the cleaning and maintenance debridement of wounds. Low levels of ultrasound energy may be carried to the wound by the saline mist. These are Class II devices.

Wound imaging devices include the following:

- Wound measurement and documentation systems (Class II)
- Wound autofluorescence imaging devices: used to view autofluorescence images from skin wounds after exposure to excitation light (Class II, or Class I via De Novo)
- Wound imaging systems for study of blood flow in the microcirculation (Class II)

ADDITIONAL SOURCES OF INFORMATION

Submissions for medical devices contain confidential and proprietary information. However, public databases provide summaries of the material provided for Class II and Class III devices that have been cleared or approved, respectively.

Class II device 510(k) summaries, available in the searchable 510(k) Premarket Notification Web site, provide the technical specifications of the device, the Intended Use/IFU, a comparison to the specifications and the Intended Use/IFU of the predicate device or devices, and a summary of performance data provided in support of the device.[20] Devices cleared under 510(k) begin with the letter K, followed by a 6-digit number; the first 2 digits indicate the year the device was submitted for review.

De Novo submissions can be searched in the de novo database.[21] A complete (and searchable) list of De Novos granted is also available online with links to the Classification Order and the Decision Summary.[22]

Class III devices can be found by searching the PMA database.[23] PMA approvals begin with the letter P, followed by a 6-digit number; the first 2 digits indicate the year the device was submitted for review. The database will provide links to the Approval Order, which will include any required postapproval activities, such postapproval studies; to the Summary of Safety and Effectiveness Data; to any supplements of approved changes; and to the approved labeling, which includes the Intended Use, IFU, warnings/precautions, preclinical and clinical data provided, instructions for use, and patient information, if relevant.[24]

Medical devices remain under FDA regulation and oversight after they are cleared or approved. Under the Medical Device Reporting (MDR) regulation, device manufacturers who have received complaints of device malfunctions, serious injuries, or deaths associated with medical devices are required to notify FDA of the incident. User facilities (eg, hospitals, nursing homes) are also required to report suspected medical device-related deaths and injuries to the FDA. Adverse events data from MDRs can be found on the Manufacturer and User Facility Device Experience database.[25] MDRs can help monitor device performance and identify safety concerns related to a particular device or technology. Although MDRs are a valuable source of information, this passive surveillance system has limitations; the incidence or prevalence of an adverse event cannot be determined from this reporting system alone because of underreporting of events, inaccuracies in reports, lack of verification that the device caused the reported event, and lack of information about frequency of device use.

DISCLOSURE

The authors have nothing to disclose.

This article reflects the views of the authors and should not be construed to represent FDA's views or policies.

REFERENCES

1. US Food and Drug Administration: medical device overview. Available at: www.fda.gov/industry/regulated-products/medical-device-overview. Accessed April 4, 2021.
2. Office of combination products, U.S. Food & Drug Administration. Available at: https://www.fda.gov/about-fda/office-clinical-policy-and-programs/office-combination-products. Accessed April 19, 2021.
3. Frequently asked questions about combination products. Available at: https://www.fda.gov/combination-products/about-combination-products/frequently-asked-questions-about-combination-products#CP. Accessed May 11, 2021.
4. Code of federal regulations 21CFR 801.4. Available at: www.accessdata.fda.gov/scripts/cdrh/cfdocs/cfcfr/CFRSearch.cfm?FR=801.4. Accessed March 18, 2022.
5. Code of federal regulations 21CFR 814.20. Available at: www.accessdata.fda.gov/scripts/cdrh/cfdocs/cfcfr/CFRSearch.cfm?fr=814.20. Accessed March 18, 2022.
6. Code of federal regulations 21CFR 860.3. Available at: www.accessdata.fda.gov/scripts/cdrh/cfdocs/cfcfr/cfrsearch.cfm?fr=860.3. Accessed March 18, 2022.
7. Medical device exemptions 510(k) and GMP requirements: part 878 - general and plastic surgery devices. Available at: www.accessdata.fda.gov/scripts/cdrh/cfdocs/cfpcd/315.cfm?GMPPart=878#start. Accessed March 18, 2022.
8. Federal Food, Drug, and Cosmetic Act (FD&C Act). Available at: www.fda.gov/regulatory-information/federal-food-drug-and-cosmetic-act-fdc-act/fdc-act-chapter-v-drugs-and-devices#Part_A. Accessed April 6, 2021.
9. Goldman L. Effects of new laser systems on the skin. Arch Dermatol 1973;108(3):385–90.
10. Medical device accessories – describing accessories and classification pathways. Available at: www.fda.gov/media/90647/download. Accessed April 8, 2021.
11.. 878.4635 Sunlamp products and ultraviolet lamps intended for use in sunlamp products. Available at: https://ecfr.federalregister.gov/current/title-21/chapter-I/subchapter-H/part-878/subpart-E/section-878.4635. Accessed March 18, 2022.
12.. General and Plastic Surgery Devices: Reclassification of Ultraviolet Lamps for Tanning, Henceforth To Be Known as Sunlamp Products and Ultraviolet Lamps Intended for Use in Sunlamp Products. Federal Register, 2014;79:31205-31214 Section 105, Rules and RegulationsDeoartment of Health and Human Services. Available at: https://

www.govinfo.gov/content/pkg/FR-2014-06-02/pdf/ 2014-12546.pdf. Accessed March 18, 2022.

13. FDA-approved dermal fillers. 2020. Available at: www.fda.gov/medical-devices/aesthetic-cosmetic-devices/fda-approved-dermal-fillers. Accessed April 6, 2021.

14. FDA executive summary general issues panel meeting on dermal fillers March 23, 2021. 2021. Available at: www.fda.gov/media/146870/download. Accessed April 6, 2021.

15. FDA warns against use of injectable silicone for body contouring and enhancement: FDA safety communication. 2017. Available at: www.fda.gov/ medical-devices/safety-communications/fda-warns-against-use-injectable-silicone-body-contouring-and-enhancement-fda-safety-communication. Accessed April 6, 2021.

16. FDA premarket approval (PMA) database. Available at: www.accessdata.fda.gov/scripts/cdrh/cfdocs/ cfPMA/pma.cfm. Accessed April 6, 2021.

17. Approved uses of dermal fillers. 2020. Available at: www.fda.gov/medical-devices/aesthetic-cosmetic-devices/dermal-fillers-soft-tissue-fillers. Accessed April 6, 2021.

18. Dermal fillers (soft tissue fillers). Available at: www. fda.gov/medical-devices/aesthetic-cosmetic-

devices/dermal-fillers-soft-tissue-fillers. Accessed Aptil 6, 2021.

19. FDA executive summary: classification of wound dressings combined with drugs. 2016. Available at: www.fda.gov/media/100005/download. Accessed March 18, 2022.

20. 510(k) premarket notification database. Available at: www.accessdata.fda.gov/scripts/cdrh/cfdocs/ cfpmn/pmn.cfm. Accessed March 18, 2022.

21. Device Classification Under Section 513(f)(2)(de novo). Available at: www.accessdata.fda.gov/ scripts/cdrh/cfdocs/cfpmn/denovo.cfm. Accessed March 18, 2022.

22. Evaluation of automatic class III designation (de novo) summaries. Available at: www.fda.gov/about-fda/cdrh-transparency/evaluation-automatic-class-iii-designation-de-novo-summaries. Accessed March 18, 2022.

23. Premarket Approval (PMA) Database.

24. Chang CJ, Ashar BS, Marquart LN. The US Food and Drug Administration's approach for safe innovation of medical devices in dermatology. JAMA Dermatol 2018;154(3):261–3.

25. MAUDE - manufacturer and user facility device experience. Available at: www.accessdata.fda. gov/scripts/cdrh/cfdocs/cfmaude/search.cfm. Accessed March 18, 2022.

Regulation of Cosmetics in the United States

Linda M. Katz, MD, MPH*, Kathleen M. Lewis, JD[1], Susan Spence, PhD, Nakissa Sadrieh, PhD

KEYWORDS

- Cosmetics • Personal care products • Food and Drug Administration • Regulatory • Adulteration
- Misbranding • Toxicity • Safety

KEY POINTS

- Under the Food, Drug, and Cosmetic Act (FD&C Act), cosmetic ingredients and products are not subject to premarket approval, with the exception of color additives. Cosmetics must not be adulterated or misbranded.
- FDA has regulations for cosmetic labeling and specific ingredients. In addition, cosmetic labeling must adhere to the FD&C Act and Fair Packaging and Labeling Act.
- The law does not require cosmetic labeling to have premarket approval. However, there are limits to cosmetic labeling claims.
- Manufacturers and other responsible parties are responsible for ensuring that products they are selling are safe under the intended conditions of use.

INTRODUCTION

The scope of cosmetic products regulated in the United States, as well as abroad, is large, and most consumers use more than 1 cosmetic product every day. It has been estimated that women, on average, use 12 cosmetic products daily versus 6 products for men.[1] Examples of such products include moisturizers, hair care products, makeup, shaving preparations, nail polishes, perfumes, some toothpastes, mouthwashes, face and body cleaners, and deodorants. It has been estimated that the annual sales of all cosmetic products in the United States is greater than $89.5 billion.[2]

The original Food and Drug Act of 1906, also known as "The Pure Food and Drug Act," did not include cosmetics (although it did include color additives for foods and drugs). During that historic era, obvious makeup was not considered "respectable"; lotions and creams were marketed to enhance natural beauty, and shampoos, lotions, creams, and even makeup were often homemade. None were regulated, and some were even considered dangerous. For example, Laird's Bloom of Youth, circa 1860, was used for the complexion and skin but was found to have dangerous lead content. Attempts to include cosmetics in the 1906 Act failed because cosmetics were (1) a small part of the economy; (2) used by a limited segment of the population; and (3) viewed as unnecessary.

As outside influences came to bear toward the 1920s, such as the film industry's use of cosmetics and women entering the workforce, changes began to be seen in commerce, including direct sale of cosmetics in retail stores like "Five & Ten" (cent) stores and in beauty salons. Concern for the regulation of foods, drugs, and cosmetics continued into the 1930s. Two perfectly legal cosmetic products at the time, Koremlu and Lash Lure, brought widespread attention and publicity to the problem of unregulated cosmetics. Koremlu was a depilatory containing thallium acetate, a rat poison. Its use caused baldness, polyneuropathy, and paralysis. Lash Lure was an aniline dye for eyelashes, the use of which caused severe dermatitis, conjunctival edema, corneal ulceration, and blindness. In the early 1930s, several adverse

Office of Cosmetics and Colors, Center for Food Safety and Nutrition, US Food and Drug Administration, 5001 Campus Drive, HFS-100, College Park, MD 20740, USA
[1] Now retired; c/o linda.katz@fda.hhs.gov
* Corresponding author.
E-mail address: linda.katz@fda.hhs.gov

Dermatol Clin 40 (2022) 307–318
https://doi.org/10.1016/j.det.2022.02.006
0733-8635/22/Published by Elsevier Inc.

events related to these products were reported in the *Journal of American Medical Association*.[3,4] These included 1 case of permanent blindness in a prominent socialite and 1 death associated with the use of Lash Lure. These injuries and more led to Congress to authorize the inclusion of cosmetics in consumer legislation, which culminated in the Federal Food, Drug, and Cosmetic Act of 1938 (FD&C Act or the Act).[5]

LAWS AND REGULATIONS
Laws

The Food and Drug Administration's (FDA) authority over cosmetics comes from the following laws: (1) the FD&C Act of 1938, which defined cosmetics and stipulated FDA's authority; (2) the Color Additive Amendments (1960), which provides for the regulation of color additives, including the commodities in which they may be used; and (3) the Fair Packaging and Labeling Act (FPLA, 1966), which provides for labeling regulations of cosmetic products.

Under section 201(i) of the FD&C Act (21 U.S.C. 321), cosmetics are defined as articles, other than soap, intended for cleansing, beautifying, promoting attractiveness, and altering appearance. Under section 201(g) (1) of the FD&C Act (21 U.S.C. 321), drugs are defined as articles intended for the diagnosis, cure, mitigation, treatment, or prevention of disease, as well as articles, other than food, affecting the structure or any function of the body of humans or animals.[6] Some products are considered cosmetic-drug products and are subject to regulations for both product categories (**Table 1**). Soaps, depending on processing and indications, may be regulated as a cosmetic: if the intent is for cleansing or beautifying, as a drug; if it is an antiseptic or has antimicrobial claims, or by the Consumer Product Safety Commission (CPSC) if it is a traditional soap made primarily from fats and alkalis.[7]

Of note, there is no regulatory definition of "cosmeceuticals" or "personal care products," both of which are terms used by industry and others. The former has been used to describe cosmetics that do something more. However, once structure and function claims are made, the products may be classified as drugs or drug cosmetics depending on the claims. The latter term, "personal care products," encompasses cosmetics, over-the-counter drugs, some devices, and some products regulated by CPSC.

Within the FD&C Act, several laws prohibit placing cosmetics or any product that FDA regulates into interstate commerce if that product is adulterated or misbranded (**Table 2**). This means that nearly everyone involved in cosmetics, including manufacturers, packers, distributors, and retailers, is responsible for assuring that he or she is not dealing in products that are adulterated or misbranded, even if someone else caused the adulteration or misbranding in the first place. If a product is introduced into interstate commerce or received in interstate commerce, the party marketing the product is responsible. The law applies to components and packaging as well as to finished products.[8]

Adulteration

Under section 601 of the FD&C Act (21 U.S.C. 361), a cosmetic is deemed to be adulterated if it bears or contains a poisonous or deleterious substance that may render it injurious to users under the conditions of use prescribed on the product labeling or under conditions that are customary or usual, with the exception of coal tar dyes; if it consists in whole or in part of any filthy, putrid, or decomposed substance; if it has been prepared, packed, or held under insanitary conditions whereby it may have become contaminated with filth, or whereby it may have been rendered injurious to health; if its container is composed, in whole or in part, of any poisonous or deleterious substance that may render the contents injurious to health; or if it is not a hair dye and it is, or it bears or contains, a color additive that is unsafe within the meaning of section 721(a) of the FD&C Act. Section 721(a) of the FD&C Act (21 U.S.C. 379(a)) states the circumstances under which color additives are deemed unsafe.[8]

The term "coal tar dyes" dates back to the time when these coloring materials were byproducts of the coal industry. Today, most are made from petroleum, but the original name is still used. The "exception of coal tar dyes" means that FDA cannot take action against coal tar hair dye on the basis that it is or contains a poisonous or deleterious ingredient that may make it harmful to consumers, as long as the label includes a special caution statement and as long as the product comes with adequate directions for consumers to do a skin test before they dye their hair. In addition, coal tar hair dyes, unlike color additives in general, do not need FDA approval according to the language of the FD&C Act.[9]

Misbranding

Under section 602 of the FD&C Act (21 U.S.C. 362) a cosmetic is misbranded: (1) if its labeling is false or misleading in any particular, or, if the cosmetic is in package form; (2) if the label is missing the name and place of business of the manufacturer,

Table 1
Cosmetics versus drugs, and their regulatory differences

FDA Classification	Definitions	Regulatory Differences	Some Examples
Cosmetics	FD&C Act, Section 201(i) Articles intended for: Cleansing Beautifying Promoting attractiveness Altering appearance	*No pre-market approval* required *No pre-market clearance* of safety or efficacy GMP: Voluntary • *No* mandatory records access • *No* mandatory establishment or product registration • Adverse events reporting is *not* mandatory Must not be adulterated or misbranded	Moisturizers, other skin preparations Hair care, hair dyes, hair straighteners Makeup, nail polishes Shaving preparations Perfumes Some toothpastes, mouthwashes Face and body cleansers, deodorants Tattoos (permanent and temporary)
Over-the-counter drugs	FD&C Act, Section 201(g) (1) Articles intended for disease: Diagnosis Cure Mitigation Treatment Prevention Affecting the structure or any function of the body of humans or animals	*Pre-market approval* or monograph Safety and efficacy Subject to GMP by regulation • Mandatory Records access • Establishments and products *must* be registered • Serious adverse events *must* be reported to the FDA Must be safe and effective	Antiredness or sunburn products Antiaging or antiwrinkle products Acne, eczema, psoriasis medications Topically applied hormones Wart removers Most skin bleaching products Antiseptics and antimicrobials Antiperspirants Hair growth/loss products
Cosmetic-drug combination products	Meet both definitions	Regulated as drugs	Antimicrobial cleanser Antidandruff shampoo Anticaries toothpaste Antiperspirant-deodorant

packer, or distributor; (3) if an accurate statement of the quantity contents in terms of weight, measure, or numerical count is not listed; (4) if any word, statement, or other information required by or under authority of the FD&C Act is not prominently placed with conspicuousness and in such a way as it is likely to be read and understood by an ordinary individual under customary conditions of purchase and use; (5) if the container is made, formed, or filled as to be misleading; or (6) if it is a color additive, unless the packaging or labeling conforms to the packaging and labeling requirements applicable to color additives contained in the regulations issued under section 721 of the FD&C Act (21 U.S.C. 379e(a)).[8] However, this requirement does not apply to packages of color additives used for cosmetics that are marketed and intended for use only in or on hair dyes (coal tar dyes), which are exempt.

Under section 201(n) of the FD&C Act, a determination that labeling is "misleading" includes considering both what the label says and what it fails to reveal. In other words, if an article is alleged to be misbranded because the labeling or advertising is misleading, then a determination takes into account (among other things) not only representations made or suggested by statement, word, design, device, or any combination but also the extent to which the labeling or advertising fails to reveal material facts represented, or required, or consequences related to material facts based on use of the article as purported on the labeling or under customary or usual use of the article.[8]

Table 2
Hazards prohibited under the Food, Drug, and Cosmetic Act

Adulterated cosmetics	Misbranded cosmetics
• Harmful or injurious under labeled or customary conditions of use • Consists of filthy substance • Prepared, packed, or held under unsanitary conditions and contaminated or rendered injurious • Container is composed of poisonous substances rendering the product injurious • Unapproved color additive *"Coal Tar Hair Dye Exemption" (Sec. 601(a))	• False or misleading labeling or does not contain all required information • Unlabeled packaging • Labeling improperly placed or inconspicuous • Misleading container • Color additive (other than hair dye) does not conform to applicable regulations under section 721 of the FD&C Act • Noncompliant packaging (does not comply with Poison Prevention Packaging Act of 1970) • Under FPLA: does not contain ingredient declaration so consumers can make informed purchase decisions

Under section 10(a) of the FPLA (15 U.S.C. 1459(a)), a consumer commodity (as it applies to FDA-regulated products) is any food, drug, device, or cosmetic (as defined by the FD&C Act) and any other article, product, or commodity of any kind or class that is customarily produced or distributed for sale through retail sales agencies or for consumption by individuals, or use by individuals for personal care or in the performance of services ordinarily rendered in the household and that are usually consumed or expended in the course of consumption or use. A consumer commodity is defined by the way it is marketed, not by the way it is labeled by FPLA. Therefore, labeling a product with "For Professional Use Only," for example, will not keep the product from being considered a consumer commodity.[10]

In addition, under section 7(a) of the FPLA (15 U.S.C. 1456(a)), when a cosmetic is marketed in violation of the FPLA or any implementing regulations, it is considered misbranded. Cosmetics offered for sale as consumer commodities need label information, such as the product's identity, statement of use, directions of use, and applicable warnings. The FPLA allows for the implementation of regulations for required label information, ingredient declaration, and prevention of deceptive packaging.[8]

Regulations

The FD&C Act and FPLA contain provisions that define FDA's level of control over cosmetic products. To implement these statutes, FDA develops, publishes, and implements regulations and guidance. The Federal Register (FR) is the official daily publication for rules, proposed rules, and notices of guidances. Proposed rules are initially published in the FR for public comment. Final regulations are published in the FR and subsequently placed or codified into the Code of Federal Regulations (CFR) on an annual basis. Generally, regulations have an effective date and a compliance date, specifying when the regulation is in effect and when compliance is expected. FDA often specifies different compliance dates depending on the size of a business, with small businesses getting more time.

The CFR is a codification of the rules that were published in the FR by the federal government. It is divided into 50 titles that represent broad areas subject to federal regulation.[11] FDA's cosmetic regulations are found in 21 CFR parts 700 through 740, describing the general provisions, requirements for specific cosmetic products, cosmetic labeling in general and for specific ingredients, warning statements, and the Voluntary Cosmetic Registration Program (VCRP). FDA's color additive regulations are found in 21 CFR parts 70, 71, 73, 74, 80, 81, and 82.[12] Declaration of color additives on cosmetic labels is addressed in 21 CFR part 701.3.

All color additives must be approved by FDA before being used in cosmetics or any other FDA-regulated product. There must be a regulation specifically addressing a substance's use as a color additive, with specifications, and, as necessary, restrictions. In addition to approval, many color additives must meet the requirements for identity and specifications stated in the CFR.[13,14] In contrast, the final formulation of a cosmetic product and its ingredients does not have premarket approval, but the product and its ingredients must not be adulterated or misbranded. As noted above, this means that cosmetics cannot contain hazardous or deleterious material (section 601 of the FD&C Act; 21 U.S.C. 361), be packaged in such a way as to be misleading or be harmful under customary or usual conditions of use (section 602 of the FD&C Act/21 U.S.C. 362; and FPLA sections 1453-1456/15 U.S.C. 1453 and 1454).[8] Furthermore, cosmetic products cannot be misbranded; this means that the labeling must be accurate, with clear directions and instructions for use, must contain appropriate warning statements, and must adhere to the requirements in the above laws. Under the FD&C Act, it is the responsibility of the manufacturer and other responsible parties to ensure that the products that they are selling are safe under the intended conditions of use (**Table 3**). How this is done is left up to the manufacturers, but often they rely on data generated from clinical trials, published literature, or other sources. Cosmetic products not adhering to the laws and regulations are subject to FDA enforcement action.

Cosmetic Labeling Claims

The law does not require cosmetic labeling to have FDA approval before cosmetic products go on the

---

Table 3
Some regulatory considerations for manufacturing and marketing a cosmetic product in the United States

Component	Considerations (References)
Ingredients	• Must not be on FDA's prohibited or restricted list[20] • Must not be adulterated, which means among other things that they should not contain harmful or deleterious ingredients or contaminants[8,36] • Must be safe (toxicology tests or literature)[24] • Color additives (other than "coal tar dyes") must be FDA approved for the intended use. In addition, some color additives must be batch-tested and certified[13]
Manufacturing	• FDA guidance for GMP[25] provides useful information about facilities and equipment and their maintenance, as well as information about trained personnel, ingredient sourcing, storage, and production practices, laboratory controls, labeling, good record-keeping,[37] and how to avoid contamination of the product with filth and microbial contamination both during and after manufacture[38] • Compliance with FDA enforcement actions, and remediations when indicated by law[34,39]
Packaging	• Must not be made, filled, or labeled in a misleading way • Must be conspicuously, truthfully, and accurately labeled in plain English with the name of the product; a representation of its intended use; the net quantity of contents; name and place of business of the manufacturer or packer, or distributor; an ingredient declaration in decreasing order of predominance; directions for safe use; any required warning statements; and other features consistent with regulations[10,40] • Warning labels are required for "coal tar dyes," cosmetic aerosols, foaming bath products, feminine deodorant sprays, and products whose safety has not been substantiated[10] • Labeling should be limited to cosmetic claims, not drug claims unless drug laws and regulations have been followed[6]
Overall	• It is against the law to market a cosmetic that is harmful to consumers when they use it according to the labeled directions, or in the customary or expected way • Resources for industry and for small business manufacturers can be found at FDA Web sites[41,42] • Voluntary registration of the product and firm can be done in FDA's Voluntary Cosmetic Registration Program[23] • Voluntary reporting of any adverse events or consumer complaints is encouraged[27,28]

market, and FDA does not have a list of approved or accepted claims for cosmetics. However, there are regulatory requirements that apply to cosmetic labeling claims.

In general, a product label consists of a principal display panel and several side panels upon which product information is placed. A product's principal display panel must state the common or usual name of the product (or an appropriately descriptive name or, when the cosmetic's nature is obvious, a fanciful name understood by the public to identify the cosmetic) (21 CFR 701.11(b) (1) and (2)), provide an appropriate illustration or vignette representing the intended cosmetic use (21 CFR 701.11(a) (3)), and accurately state the net quantity of its contents (21 CFR 701.13).[10] Side or back information panels typically state the name and address of the distributor (21 CFR 701.12), a list of ingredients in plain English and in decreasing order of predominance (21 CFR 701.3), and directions for safe use of the product. If required by law, they should also include conspicuous warning statements (21 CFR 40 (1) and (2)). If the product is imported, the country of origin must be identified in English (21 CFR 701.2).[10]

Under the law, information on cosmetic labeling, including claims, must be truthful and not misleading. In addition, if a product is intended to be used for purposes such as treating or preventing disease, or affecting the structure or function of the body, including the skin, it is a drug according to the law, and it must meet the requirements for drugs, even if it affects the appearance, the cosmetic portion of the label. For example, anti-dandruff shampoos are such products, because the "anti-dandruff" claim, which is designed to treat a condition, is a drug, whereas the "shampoo" claim for cleansing is a cosmetic claim.

Because FDA does not have the authority to approve claims before cosmetics go on the market, cosmetics with claims that go beyond what the law permits may occur. FDA, however, monitors cosmetics on the market and can take action against companies that break the laws we enforce. For example, FDA has issued warning letters to cosmetic firms that have made unapproved drug claims for products marketed as cosmetics.

In addition, although FDA regulates cosmetic labeling claims, the Federal Trade Commission regulates advertising claims.[15]

Banned Ingredients in the United States

With the exception of color additives and a few prohibited ingredients, a cosmetic manufacturer may use almost any raw material as a cosmetic ingredient and market the product without approval from FDA. Although it is against the law to use any ingredient that makes a cosmetic harmful when used as intended, FDA has regulations that specifically prohibit or restrict the use of the following ingredients in cosmetics: bithionol, mercury compounds, vinyl chloride, certain halogenated salicylanilides, zirconium complexes in aerosol cosmetics, chloroform, methylene chloride, and chlorofluorocarbon propellants (21 CFR part 700).[16,17]

In addition, cosmetics may not be manufactured from, processed with, or otherwise contain, certain prohibited cattle materials. These materials include material from nonambulatory cattle, material from cattle not inspected and passed, or mechanically separated beef. This is to protect consumers against contracting bovine spongiform encephalopathy or "mad cow disease" through the use of cosmetics (21 CFR 700.27).

Color additives are permitted in cosmetics only if FDA has approved them for that intended use. In addition, some color additives may only be used if they are from batches that FDA has tested and certified (21 CFR parts 74 and 82).[13]

Several color additives approved for cosmetic use in general are not approved for use in the area of the eyes (21 CFR 70.5(a)). The "area of the eye" means the area enclosed within the circumference of the supraorbital ridge and the infraorbital ridge, including the eyebrow, the skin below the eyebrow, the eyelids and the eyelashes, and conjunctival sac of the eye, the eyeball, and the soft areolar tissue that lies within the perimeter of the infraorbital ridge (21 CFR 70.3(s)). Although there are color additives approved for use in products such as mascara and eyebrow pencils, silver nitrate was recently approved for professional use in dyeing the eyebrows or eyelashes.[14] Consumers should be aware that if color additives are not approved by FDA for use in the area of the eyes, FDA has not received, evaluated, and approved information supporting the safety of these color additives when used in this way.[18]

If a color additive is approved for use in externally applied cosmetics, it may not be used in products such as lipsticks unless the regulation specifically permits this use (21 CFR 70.3(v)). Also, the fact that a color additive is listed for any other FDA-authorized use does not mean that it may be used for injections, such as in tattooing (21 CFR 70.5(b)), unless specifically evaluated for safety in that context.[14]

If a color additive is not used according to the listing in the CFR, it is considered to be adulterated. A disclaimer is not acceptable to permit the use of an unapproved color additive.[19]

FDA often gets asked why different ingredients are prohibited in some other countries. Different countries and regions regulate cosmetics under different legal frameworks. FDA can take other countries' decisions into consideration, but can only take action within the legal and regulatory framework for cosmetics in the United States.[20,21]

DOMESTIC ACTIVITIES
Voluntary Cosmetic Registration Program

FDA's VCRP is a reporting system for use by manufacturers, packers, and distributors of cosmetic products that are in commercial distribution in the United States as defined by section 201(i) of the FD&C Act.[22] Commercial distribution of a cosmetic product means annual gross sales in excess of $1000 for that product (21 CFR 700.3(i)). Registration in VCRP does not apply to cosmetic products for professional use only, such as products used in beauty salons, spas, or skin care clinics. It also does not apply to products that are not for sale, such as hotel samples, free gifts, or "homemade" cosmetic products. Like domestic products, imported products may also voluntarily register if they are marketed in the United States. Products that are considered drugs in the United States, such as sunscreens, but that also make cosmetic claims, such as moisturizing, can be filed in the VCRP; however, if a product is either solely a drug or a drug/cosmetic product, it is subject by law to different requirements than those for products that are solely cosmetics, including requirements for product listing and establishment registration according to section 510 of the FD&C Act[23] and 21 CFR 207.

The VCRP assists FDA in carrying out its responsibility to regulate cosmetics marketed in the United States. However, because product filings and establishment registrations are not mandatory, voluntary submissions only provide FDA with an incomplete estimate of information available about cosmetic products marketed in the United States, including ingredients, their frequency of use, and the businesses engaged in their manufacture and distribution (21 CFR 720.1 and 720.2; 73 FR 76360; 69 FR 9339; 21 CFR parts 710 and 720). The VCRP is not a cosmetic approval program or a promotional tool. As previously mentioned, cosmetics are not subject to FDA premarket approval, and it is the firm's responsibility to ensure that its cosmetic products and ingredients are safe and properly labeled, in full compliance with the law. Registration of a cosmetic establishment, assignment of an establishment registration number, filing a cosmetic product, or assignment of a CPIS number does not mean that FDA has approved the firm or its products (21 CFR 710.8 and 720.9) or that a product is a cosmetic as defined in the FD&C Act. Any representation in labeling or advertising that creates an impression of official approval because of registration or possession of a registration number is considered misleading (21 CFR 710.8 and 720.9). Under section 602(a) of the FD&C Act, misleading labeling makes a cosmetic misbranded.

There are 2 parts to the VCRP filing.[23] Companies may participate in both parts of the program or only 1 part. They may also choose whether to register the establishment (Form FDA 2511), file Cosmetic Product Ingredient Statements (Form FDA 2512), or both. Specific requirements can be found on FDA's Web site.[23]

When a product is made by a contract manufacturer and distributed by a different firm, either the contract manufacturer or the distributor can enter the formulation into the VCRP, but not both. The 2 companies need to decide who will enter the formulation.

Any firm, once having filed an original cosmetic formulation, is responsible for maintaining an accurate filing with FDA for that formulation. Changes to a brand name or ingredients may be submitted within 60 days after beginning commercial distribution of the changed cosmetic product in the United States. Other changes may be submitted within 1 year after such changes occur (21 CFR 720.6). Any firm, once having filed a cosmetic formulation (Form FDA 2512), should discontinue it within 180 days after the product is no longer in commercial distribution (21 CFR 720.6).

Information from the VCRP database has been used by the Cosmetic Ingredient Review (CIR) to assist the CIR Expert Panel in establishing their priorities for assessing ingredient safety as part of their ingredient safety review. The CIR is an industry-funded panel of scientific experts who conduct evaluation of the safety of individual ingredients used in cosmetic products.[24] The CIR was established in 1976 by the Cosmetic, Toiletry and Fragrance Association (now the Personal Care Products Council) with the goal of unbiased evaluation of the safety of individual ingredients used in cosmetic products. To achieve this goal, the CIR (1) identifies cosmetic ingredients for review; (2) drafts ingredient safety assessment reports; (3) facilitates discussions about cosmetic ingredient safety between the CIR Expert Panel and representatives from FDA's Office of Cosmetics and Colors (OCAC) and consumer safety groups at publicly held meetings; and (4) publishes final safety assessment reports in peer reviewed journals.

Good Manufacturing Practices

In 2013, FDA issued a draft guidance, the "Cosmetic Good Manufacturing (GMP) Guidelines/Inspection Checklist," that set forth current practices and clarified certain topic areas based on experience.[25] It is intended to assist industry and other stakeholders to identify the standards and issues that can affect the quality of cosmetic products. In addition, as part of an international harmonization effort with the International Cooperation on Cosmetic Regulations (ICCR), FDA, as well as other ICCR member jurisdictions, agreed to consider the International Organization for Standardization (ISO) standard for cosmetic GMPs (ISO 22716:2007)[26] when revising previous draft guidance. As such, we reviewed ISO 22716 and decided to incorporate, modify, or exclude specific aspects of it into our guidance based on our experience.

FDA's guidance documents, including this guidance, do not establish legally enforceable responsibilities. Instead, guidances describe FDA's current thinking on a topic and should be viewed only as recommendations, unless specific regulatory or statutory requirements are cited. The use of the word *should* in FDA guidances means that something is suggested or recommended, but not required.[25]

Adverse Event Reporting

Reporting of cosmetic adverse events and product complaints by health care providers, industry, and consumers is voluntary in the United States. Reporting is an important way that FDA learns about potential issues with cosmetic products. Consumers, cosmetic professionals, manufacturers, and health care professionals can notify FDA if they experience or learn of problems that they think arise from use of cosmetic products. These include (1) a reaction after using a cosmetic, such as a rash, redness, burn, hair loss, headache, infection, illness, or any other unexpected reaction, whether or not it required medical treatment; and (2) a problem with a cosmetic product, such as bad smell, color change, other sign of contamination, or foreign material in the product. In the case of a reaction or problem with a cosmetic product, consumers are advised to stop using the product, contact their health care provider, and then report the problem to FDA. FDA keeps all personal information confidential (21 CFR 20.63).

Problems about cosmetics can be reported to FDA in any of 3 ways[27,28]: by completing an electronic Voluntary MedWatch form online,[29] by completing a paper Voluntary Medwatch form,[30] or by calling an FDA Consumer Complaint Coordinator in their area if they wish to speak directly to a person about their problem[31] (**Box 1**).

The Center for Food Safety and Applied Nutrition (CFSAN) Adverse Event Reporting System (CAERS) is a database[32] that contains information on adverse event and product complaint reports submitted to FDA about foods, dietary supplements, and cosmetics. CAERS data, without personal identifying information, are available online and can be searched by the general public. Cosmetic adverse event reports received voluntarily from consumers, health care professionals, cosmetics professionals, and manufacturers are entered into CAERS. These reports can include minor to major medical events, but also complaints about off-smell or off-color of a product, defective packaging, and other nonmedical issues. FDA receives some adverse event and product complaint reports directly from health care professionals and consumers or their representatives (such as family members, lawyers, and others). Health care professionals and consumers may also report adverse events to the products' manufacturers. If a manufacturer receives a serious adverse event report related to a cosmetic product, the manufacturer may forward the report to CAERS, but it is not a legal requirement.

FDA uses CAERS to look for new safety concerns that might be related to a marketed product, to evaluate a manufacturer's compliance to reporting requirements, and to respond to outside requests for information. The reports in CAERS are evaluated by clinical reviewers in the CFSAN who monitor the safety of consumer products. If a potential safety concern is identified in CAERS, further evaluation is performed. Based on an evaluation of the potential safety concern, FDA may take compliance or regulatory action or actions to address product safety, communicate new safety information to the public, or remove a product from the market. FDA may not take action on every report, but the Agency does check all reports for trending purposes, which will help to determine if action is necessary to protect the public health.

As noted above, because reporting of adverse events by consumers, health care professionals, cosmetic professionals, and manufacturers is not mandatory, this often means that FDA is receiving data from only a small fraction of consumers who may potentially be experiencing problems with a product. Also, the reports submitted to FDA vary in the quality and reliability of the information provided. Some reports do not include all relevant data, such as whether an individual also has underlying medical conditions or used other cosmetic products, medications, or supplements

---

Box 1
Reporting adverse events to the Food and Drug Administration

If your patient has an infection, allergic reaction, or another adverse event that may be due to a cosmetic product or tattoo, please file a report with the FDA in any of 3 ways:

- Online MedWatch Reporting: https://www.accessdata.fda.gov/scripts/medwatch/
- MedWatch Paper Form: https://www.fda.gov/safety/medical-product-safety-information/medwatch-forms-fda-safety-reporting
- Regional Complaint Coordinators: http://www.fda.gov/Safety/ReportaProblem/ConsumerComplaint Coordinators

Reports to FDA should include the following information:

- About the person affected:
  - Name and contact information (address, telephone number, and e-mail address)
  - Age, gender, and ethnicity
- About the product:
  - Name of the product and manufacturer
  - Product codes or identifying marks on the label or container (Note: do not discard the product packaging and labeling. They provide information that will help FDA investigate the problem.)
  - When and where the product was purchased
- About the problem
  - Description of the reaction or problem
  - Description of medical treatment provided, if any

Reports from consumers and physicians are an important means to identify hazardous products and may initiate regulatory enforcement actions.

---

at the same time. Reports may not include accurate or complete contact information for FDA to seek further information about the event, or complainants may choose not to participate in a follow-up investigation. When important information is missing from a report, it may be difficult for FDA to fully evaluate whether the product caused the adverse event or simply coincided with it. Therefore, FDA encourages consumers to use its online reporting system, which prompts them to provide appropriate information. Unless FDA follows up, the information in CAERS reports has not been scientifically or otherwise verified as to a cause-and-effect relationship and cannot be used to estimate incidence (occurrence rate) or to estimate risk.

The most frequently reported adverse events among cosmetic products are for hair care (including shampoos, conditioners, hair smoothing products, and hair dyes) and skin care products.[33] In addition, FDA receives more reports for leave-on then rinse-off products.

Recalls

FDA regulations define a "recall" as a firm's removal or correction of a marketed product that FDA considers to be in violation of the laws that it administers and against which FDA would initiate legal action, such as seizure (21 CFR 7.3(g)).

FDA has no authority under the FD&C Act to order a recall of a cosmetic, although it can request that a firm voluntarily recall a product.[34] FDA does, however, monitor the progress of a recall through the firm's status reports and FDA's own auditing and evaluate the health hazard and assign classification to indicate the degree of hazard posed by the recalled product (with class 1 being the greatest hazard and class 3 being the least hazard). FDA ensures that the public is notified when necessary, and it publishes general recall information in a weekly Enforcement Report.

In addition to the corrective actions of removing a violative product from the market and either destroying it or bringing it into compliance, firms should take the kind of corrective actions that prevent a similar problem from occurring in the future. That is, they should determine the cause of the violation, identify what to change to keep the problem from reoccurring, and then implement the change.[34]

INTERNATIONAL ACTIVITIES

CFSAN, in coordination with others at FDA, engages in several international activities relevant to cosmetic products. These have included bilateral discussions with a variety of different countries covering numerous issues. One of OCAC's most significant efforts had been the establishment of the International Cooperation on Cosmetics Regulation (ICCR) in 2007 as an offshoot of its predecessor, Cosmetic Harmonization and International Cooperation (CHIC), consisting of regulators from Canada, the European Union, Japan, and the United States. CHIC was established as a quadrilateral series of consultations to develop communications regarding international regulatory schemes and to seek areas of commonality for regulatory alignment (vs single global structure). In 2006, after much discussion, the group was reestablished as ICCR[35] with the goal of removing regulatory obstacles among regions, minimizing obstacles to international trade, while maintaining the highest level of consumer protection, while at the same time envisioning the possibility of future changes in structure and schedule to allow for greater inclusiveness and outreach to new jurisdictions and stakeholders (including industry, academia, and nongovernment organizations). A voluntary consensus model was established based on some of the preexisting governmental harmonization groups, such as the International Council for Harmonization of Technical Requirements for Pharmaceuticals for Human Use, with integral industry involvement. Topics of interest and relevance for the cosmetics sector have included allergens, alternatives to animal testing, integrated strategies for safety assessments, microbiome, nanotechnology, trace elements, and preservatives.

SUMMARY

Cosmetic products have continued to develop and grow in importance as a commodity globally. Cosmetics are no longer viewed as "just makeup" but have expanded to include many more product categories, many of which rely or purport to rely on innovative technologies since cosmetics was added to the FD&C Act in 1938. As the world in general has become "smaller," so, too, is the importance of communication not only within our jurisdiction but also internationally to see where collaboration in research and regulations are needed to develop safer products that can be used by all consumers.

Just as cosmetics has grown in types of products and where/how they are marketed, the regulation of cosmetics must keep pace, within the United States and internationally. Because of innovative technologies and new ingredients, such as nanoparticles, cannabidiol, and microbiotics,

regulations for cosmetics should be reviewed and updated to meet the changing technology of the twenty-first century.

This is a brief glimpse into the world of cosmetics, but the story continues, as the United States considers modernization of the cosmetics regulations. It is unclear what impact this will have on industry and the world at large.

CLINICS CARE POINTS

- Cosmetic products must not be adulterated or misbranded for safe use. Adverse events may occur with the use of any cosmetic product.
- Reporting of these adverse events is critical to FDA evaluating product safety and communicating information to consumers.
- Registration of cosmetic products helps FDA to know what is being sold and how to advise manufacturers of potential issues that may impact safety.

DISCLOSURE

All authors are/were employed by the US government and report no conflicts of interest.

REFERENCES

1. Harvard Women's Health Watch. Toxic beauty: are your personal care products putting your health at risk?. 2020. Available at: https://www.health.harvard.edu/womens-health/toxic-beauty. Accessed February 17, 2021.
2. Ridder M. Retail sales of beauty and personal care products, U.S. 2016-2019. 2020. Available at: https://www.statista.com/topics/1008/cosmetics-industry. Accessed December 2, 2020.
3. JAMA Bureau of Investigation. Koremlu: a dangerous depilatory containing thallium acetate. JAMA 1931; 96:629–31. Available at: https://jamanetwork.com/journals/jama/fullarticle/249787. Accessed February 17, 2021.
4. Gasch AT. Paraphenylenediamine: toxic beauty past and present. 2017. Available at: https://www.aao.org/senior-ophthalmologists/scope/article/lash-lure-paraphenylenediamine-toxic-beauty. Accessed February 17, 2021.
5. US Food and Drug Administration. Federal Food, Drug, and Cosmetic Act (FD&C Act). 2018. Available at: https://www.fda.gov/regulatory-information/laws-enforced-fda/federal-food-drug-and-cosmetic-act-fdc-act. Accessed February 17, 2021.

6. US Food and Drug Administration. Is it a cosmetic, a drug, or both? (Or is it soap?. 2020. Available at: https://www.fda.gov/cosmetics/cosmetics-laws-regulations/it-cosmetic-drug-or-both-or-it-soap. Accessed February 17, 2021.

7. US Consumer Product Safety Commission. Soap business guidance. Available at: https://www.cpsc.gov/Soap. Accessed February 17, 2021.

8. US Food and Drug Administration. Key legal concepts for cosmetics industry: interstate commerce, adulterated, and misbranded. 2020. Available at: https://www.fda.gov/cosmetics/cosmetics-laws-regulations/key-legal-concepts-cosmetics-industry-interstate-commerce-adulterated-and-misbranded. Accessed February 17, 2021.

9. US Food and Drug Administration. Hair dyes 2020. Available at: https://www.fda.gov/cosmetics/cosmetic-products/hair-dyes. Accessed February 17, 2021.

10. US Food and Drug Administration. Cosmetics labeling guide. 2020. Available at: https://www.fda.gov/cosmetics/cosmetics-labeling-regulations/cosmetics-labeling-guide. Accessed February 17, 2021.

11. US Food and Drug Administration. Code of federal regulations (CFR). 2018. Available at: https://www.fda.gov/medical-devices/overview-device-regulation/code-federal-regulations-cfr. Accessed February 17, 2021.

12. US Food and Drug Administration. Color additive laws, regulations, and guidance. 2019. Available at: https://www.fda.gov/industry/color-additives/color-additive-laws-regulations-and-guidance. Accessed February 17, 2021.

13. US Food and Drug Administration. Color certification FAQs. 2018. Available at: https://www.fda.gov/industry/color-certification/color-certification-faqs. Accessed February 17, 2021.

14. US Food and Drug Administration. Color additives and cosmetics: fact sheet. 2019. https://www.fda.gov/industry/color-additives-specific-products/color-additives-and-cosmetics-fact-sheet. Accessed March 15, 2022.

15. US Food and Drug Administration. Cosmetics labeling claims. 2020. Available at: https://www.fda.gov/cosmetics/cosmetics-labeling/cosmetics-labeling-claims. Accessed February 17, 2021.

16. US Government Printing Office. Electronic code of federal regulations. 2021. Available at: https://www.ecfr.gov/cgi-bin/text-idx?c=ecfr&sid=c108128827d21f2d274e894731665ef4&rgn=div6&view=text&node=21:7.0.1.2.10.2&idno=21. Accessed February 17, 2021.

17. US Food and Drug Administration. CFR-code of federal regulations title 21. 2020. https://www.accessdata.fda.gov/scripts/cdrh/cfdocs/cfcfr/CFRSearch.cfm?fr=250.250. Accessed February 17, 2021.

18. US Food and Drug Administration. Eye cosmetic safety. 2020. Available at: https://www.fda.gov/cosmetics/cosmetic-products/eye-cosmetic-safety. Accessed February 17, 2021.

19. US Food and Drug Administration. Compliance and enforcement of color additives. Available at: https://www.fda.gov/industry/color-additives/compliance-enforcement-color-additives. Accessed February 17, 2021.

20. US Food and Drug Administration. Prohibited and restricted ingredients in cosmetics. 2020. Available at: https://www.fda.gov/cosmetics/cosmetics-laws-regulations/prohibited-restricted-ingredients-cosmetics. Accessed February 17, 2021.

21. US Food and Drug Administration. Cosmetics safety Q&A: prohibited ingredients. 2020. Available at: https://www.fda.gov/cosmetics/resources-consumers-cosmetics/cosmetics-safety-qa-prohibited-ingredients. Accessed February 17, 2021.

23. US Food and Drug Administration. FD&C Act chapter V: drugs and devices. 2018. Available at: https://www.fda.gov/regulatory-information/federal-food-drug-and-cosmetic-act-fdc-act/fdc-act-chapter-v-drugs-and-devices. Accessed February 17, 2021.

22. US Food and Drug Administration. Voluntary cosmetic registration program. Available at: https://www.fda.gov/cosmetics/voluntary-cosmetic-registration-program. Accessed February 17, 2021.

24. Cosmetic ingredient review. Home page. Available at: https://cir-safety.org/. Accessed February 17, 2021.

25. US Food and Drug Administration. Draft guidance for industry: cosmetic good manufacturing practices. 2018. Available at: https://www.fda.gov/regulatory-information/search-fda-guidance-documents/draft-guidance-industry-cosmetic-good-manufacturing-practices. Accessed February 17, 2021.

26. Available at: https://www.iso.org/standard/36437.html. Accessed March 15, 2020.

27. US Food and Drug Administration. Cosmetics facts: how to report a cosmetic-related problem to FDA. 2015. Available at: https://www.fda.gov/media/92907/download. Accessed February 17, 2021.

28. US Food and Drug Administration. How to report a cosmetic related complaint. 2020. Available at: https://www.fda.gov/cosmetics/cosmetics-compliance-enforcement/how-report-cosmetic-related-complaint. Accessed February 17, 2021.

29. US Food and Drug Administration. MedWatch online voluntary reporting form. Available at: https://www.accessdata.fda.gov/scripts/medwatch/. Accessed February 17, 2021.

30. US Food and Drug Administration. MedWatch forms for FDA safety reporting. 2020. Available at: https://www.fda.gov/safety/medical-product-safety-

information/medwatch-forms-fda-safety-reporting. Accessed February 17, 2021.

31. US Food and Drug Administration. Consumer complaint coordinators. 2020. Available at: https://www.fda.gov/safety/report-problem-fda/consumer-complaint-coordinators. Accessed February 17, 2021.

32. US Food and Drug Administration. CFSAN adverse event reporting system (CAERS). 2020. Available at: https://www.fda.gov/food/compliance-enforcement-food/cfsan-adverse-event-reporting-system-caers. Accessed February 17, 2021.

33. US Food and Drug Administration. Using adverse event reports to monitor cosmetic safety. 2017. Available at: https://www.fda.gov/cosmetics/how-report-cosmetic-related-complaint/using-adverse-event-reports-monitor-cosmetic-safety. Accessed February 17, 2021.

34. US Food and Drug Administration. FDA recall policy for cosmetics. 2020. Available at: https://www.fda.gov/cosmetics/cosmetics-recalls-alerts/fda-recall-policy-cosmetics. Accessed February 17, 2021.

35. International Cooperation on Cosmetics Regulation. Home Page Available at: https://www.iccr-cosmetics.org/. Accessed February 17, 2021.

36. Potential Contaminants in Cosmetics. 2020. https://www.fda.gov/cosmetics/cosmetic-products-ingredients/potential-contaminants-cosmetics. Accessed March 9, 2021.

37. Good Manufacturing Practice (GMP) Guidelines/Inspection Checklist for Cosmetics. 2020. https://www.fda.gov/cosmetics/cosmetics-guidance-documents/good-manufacturing-practice-gmp-guidelines inspection-checklist-cosmetics. Accessed March 9, 2021.

38. Microbiological Safety and Cosmetics. 2020. Available at: https://www.fda.gov/cosmetics/potential-contaminants-cosmetics/microbiological-safety-and-cosmetics#Resources. Accessed March 9, 2021.

39. Cosmetics Compliance and Enforcement. 2020. Available at: https://www.fda.gov/cosmetics/cosmetics-compliance-enforcement. Accessed March 9, 2021.

40. Summary of Cosmetics Labeling Requirements. 2020. Available at: https://www.fda.gov/cosmetics-labeling-regulations/summary-cosmetics-labeling-requirements. Accessed March 9, 2021.

41. Resources for Industry on Cosmetics. 2020. Available at: https://www.fda.gov/cosmetics/resources-you-cosmetics/resources-industry-cosmetics. Accessed March 9, 2021.

42. Small Business and Homemade Cosmetics: Fact Sheet. 2020. Available at: https://www.fda.gov/cosmetics/resources-industry-cosmetics/small-businesses-homemade-cosmetics-fact-sheet. Accessed March 9, 2021.

Cutaneous Pharmacokinetic Approaches to Compare Bioavailability and/or Bioequivalence for Topical Drug Products

Sam G. Raney, PhD[a],*, Priyanka Ghosh, PhD[a],
Tannaz Ramezanli, Pharm D, PhD[a], Paul A. Lehman, MS[b],
Thomas J. Franz, MD[c]

KEYWORDS

- Topical • Dermatologic • Pharmacokinetics • Bioequivalence • Generics

KEY POINTS

- Extraordinary price increases for topical products, associated with insufficient competition from generics, has raised concerns about patient access to important dermatological treatments.
- The high cost of comparative clinical endpoint bioequivalence studies in patients has been a barrier to the development of topical generic products.
- The efficiency of cutaneous pharmacokinetics based bioequivalence approaches is facilitating the development of topical generics and enhancing patient access to affordable, high quality treatments.

INTRODUCTION

In simple terms, bioequivalence (BE) refers to biopharmaceutically equivalent product performance. Unlike the full evaluation of clinical safety and effectiveness that must be established when a new drug product is initially approved, the evaluation of BE involves a comparison of the test product to its reference product in a study whose fundamental scientific principles allow the clinical performance of the products to be inferred. This kind of assessment is typically relevant in two situations: when comparing a generic version of a drug product to its reference listed drug (RLD) product, or when a drug product experiences a change following approval, necessitating a demonstration of equivalent product performance despite the change.

The concept of BE exists at the intersection of science, medicine, law, and regulation. Title 21 of the US Code of Federal Regulations, Part 320 (21 CFR § 320)[1] followed by the US Food and Drug Administration (FDA) discusses bioavailability (BA) and BE requirements for drug products seeking marketing approval in the United States. These regulations evolved from the recommendations of a drug product BE study panel that was formed by the FDA's Office of Technology

a Office of Research and Standards, Office of Generic Drugs, Center for Drug Evaluation and Research, U.S. Food and Drug Administration, 10903 New Hampshire Avenue, Silver Spring, MD 20993, USA; b QPS Holdings, LLC, 3 Innovation Way, Suite 240, Newark, DE 19711, USA; c 10716 SE Forest View Lane, Happy Valley, OR 97086, USA
* Corresponding author.
E-mail address: Sameersingh.Raney@FDA.HHS.GOV

Dermatol Clin 40 (2022) 319–332
https://doi.org/10.1016/j.det.2022.02.007
0733-8635/22/Published by Elsevier Inc.

derm.theclinics.com

Assessment (OTA) in the 1970s.[2] Soon thereafter, the US Congress passed legislation that provided the framework for being able to approve generic drug products based on the results of a BE study, rather than based on clinical studies demonstrating effectiveness and safety. This legislation, the Drug Price Competition and Patent Term Restoration Act of 1984[3] (commonly known as the Hatch-Waxman Amendments) established the Abbreviated New Drug Application (ANDA) approval pathway for generic drug products and was particularly relevant for solid oral dosage forms, rather than topical or other locally acting dosage forms. Almost two decades later, the US Congress passed legislation that revised the Hatch-Waxman Amendments with Title XI of the Medicare Prescription Drug, Improvement and Modernization Act of 2003.[4] Under Title XI, "for a drug that is not intended to be absorbed into the bloodstream," the act authorized the FDA to "establish alternative, scientifically valid methods to show bioequivalence if the alternative methods are expected to detect a significant difference between the drug and the listed drug in safety and therapeutic effect." More specifically, 21 CFR § 320.24 describes several types of evidence to measure BA or establish BE.[5] Indeed, in recent decades, several test methods have been discussed and developed to evaluate topical BA and BE.[6–23] Among these, the use of pharmacokinetics (PK)-based approaches to evaluate the BA for topically applied drugs is an ideal approach by which to characterize the rate and extent to which an active ingredient becomes available at or near its site of action in the skin, and thereby, to assess the BE of test and reference topical products.[21] This is reflected in 21 CFR § 320.24, which specifies that "[an] in vivo test in humans in which the concentration of the active ingredient ... in whole blood, plasma, serum, or other appropriate biological fluid is measured as a function of time...; or [an] in vitro test that has been correlated with and is predictive of human in vivo bioavailability data" is considered to be among the most accurate, sensitive, and reproducible approach for determining the BA or BE of a product. This work provides a critical assessment of these cutaneous pharmacokinetic approaches to compare BA and/or BE for topical drug products.

IN VITRO CUTANEOUS PHARMACOKINETICS

The rationale for using an in vitro permeation test (IVPT) to support the assessment of topical BA or BE is readily apparent since it provides a simple means by which to measure the rate and extent of absorption of topically applied drugs. Use of

the model as a potential BE surrogate was discussed by regulatory and industrial scientists in 1986, and although a substantial body of literature already existed at that time on its important role in the development of topical formulations, particularly as a screening tool to evaluate the impact of vehicle modification on absorption, it was concluded that "...more experience with this application of the technology was needed."[7]

The situation is vastly different today, and IVPT is recognized by scientists worldwide as a valid technique to quantify the absorption of chemicals into and through the skin. From a regulatory perspective its application in Europe, particularly in toxicology, is relatively well established. As a result of the acceptance of Guideline OECD 428 and Guidance Document OECD 28,[22,23] which describe the procedures to be used in the conduct of IVPT, all members of the European Union (EU) accept human in vitro permeation data to assess the risk associated with dermal exposure to pesticides, biocides, cosmetic ingredients, and industrial chemicals. The European Medicines Agency (EMA) has drafted guidelines requiring the use of IVPT to characterize the performance of transdermal products as part of new marketing authorization applications, and this applies to generic applications as well.[24] In the U.S. the Environmental Protection Agency (EPA) accepts human IVPT data as part of the assessment of systemic risk for the registration of pesticides.[25–27] In 2014, the FDA first recommended an IVPT study to support a demonstration of BE in the product-specific guidance for acyclovir cream, 5%, and has since recommended IVPT studies for numerous other topical products.[28] Of all the surrogate tests available to establish topical BE, IVPT stands out as the one that has been the most studied, that appears to have the broadest application and acceptance within the scientific community, and for which the most validation data exist.

The in vitro measurement of percutaneous absorption is possible, because excised skin retains its barrier properties for several days following excision from the body. Additionally, barrier function is not damaged by freezing for many months, and then thawing, so long-term storage is possible. Conceptually, the purpose of an IVPT study and its conduct are straightforward. To quote OECD 28, "The test preparation is applied to the surface of excised skin, which is mounted in a diffusion cell. The receptor fluid, which must have an adequate capacity to solubilize the test substance, is maintained in contact with the underside of the skin from the time of application until the end of the collection of the receptor fluid. The

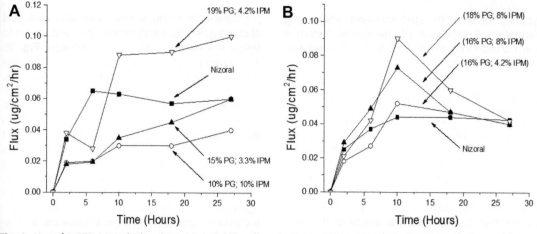

Fig. 1. Use of IVPT to match the absorption profile of a reference product (Nizoral). (*A*) Concentration of propylene glycol (PG) and isopropyl myristate (IPM) varied in 3 prototype formulations. Data suggest PG level should be between 15% and 19%. (*B*) Concentration of PG and IPM varied in 3 additional prototypes. Best match to reference product is PG = 16%, IPM = 4.2%. (*Data From* Franz TJ, Lehman PA, Raney SG. The cadaver skin absorption model and the drug development process. Pharmacopeial Forum 2008;34:1349-1356; with permission.).

test preparation remains on the skin for a specified period of time, relating to potential human exposure, and then the test preparation is removed by an appropriate cleansing procedure. The receptor fluid is sampled at time points throughout the experiment to ascertain the mass (and possibly rate) of the test substance (including any significant metabolite) passing through the skin. At the end of the study, the dislodgeable dose, the amount associated with the skin and the amount in the receptor fluid is determined. These data are necessary to calculate the total skin absorption, and allow for an estimate of the total recovery of the test substance."[23]

An example of the type of data obtained from IVPT, as well as an illustration of the sensitivity of the method, is presented in **Fig. 1**. During the development of a generic ketoconazole cream, reverse engineering failed to clearly identify the concentration of two cosolvents, propylene glycol and isopropyl myristate. Therefore, prototype formulation variants were prepared with different amounts of each of these two cosolvents, and the cutaneous PK of ketoconazole from each was compared relative to the RLD ketoconazole cream. Across 2 iterative stages of prototype formulation variation (**Fig. 1**), 6 prototype (test) formulations were evaluated, and IVPT studies were used to identify the one from which the rate and extent of ketoconazole BA best matched that of the RLD. Only 1 of the 6 was found to provide a rate and extent of absorption that closely matched that of the RLD product, and subsequent clinical evaluation confirmed its BE to the RLD product.[29]

The ultimate goal of the IVPT model system is to obtain data that are equivalent to those obtained

in vivo. To this end, several expert groups have thoroughly examined all aspects of the in vitro methodology and, for the most part, are in agreement as to several critical elements in protocol design.[23,30–32] These can be summarized as:

- Use human skin (dermatomed to $\leq$500 μ or isolated epidermis).
- Either static or flow-through chambers are acceptable.
- Maintain skin surface temperature at 32° $\pm$ 1° C.
- Verify integrity of skin barrier through measurement of ^3H_2O flux, transepidermal water loss, or electrical resistance.
- Verify drug stability in receptor solution and sample processing procedures.
- Maintain adequate solubility conditions in receptor solution (ideally, a solubility 10 times greater than needed for experimental conditions).

The latter point is critically important since many topical drugs have limited water solubility. Erroneously low absorption values can be obtained solely on the basis of inadequate receptor solubility which acts to reduce the gradient for diffusion.[33–36] The recommendation to use dermatomed skin or epidermal membranes is directed at the same potential problem. The highly aqueous dermal compartment, normally approximately 1 to 2 mm in thickness, can serve as a potential barrier to the absorption of compounds with limited water solubility. Under in vivo conditions the diffusing drug can partition into the practically infinite sink of the systemic circulation in the uppermost region of the dermis. In the in vitro (IVPT) model the drug typically traverses the epidermis and (when using dermatomed skin) part of the dermis before it can partition into the sink of a receptor solution with adequate solubility.

In Vitro/In Vivo Correlation: Percutaneous Absorption

Evidence to support use of the in vitro (IVPT) model to establish BE comes from studies of in vitro/in vivo correlation (IVIVC), and these fall into two main areas: studies that show good correlation between the amount of a compound absorbed in vitro with that absorbed in living humans, and studies that demonstrate the ability of the IVPT model to reach the same conclusion as in vivo human comparative clinical endpoint studies with respect to the BE of two drug products.

Lehman and colleagues reviewed the literature to collect data on compounds whose percutaneous absorption had been measured both in living humans and in the IVPT model.[37] Ninety-two data sets encompassing 30 compounds were collected from 30 published studies. Two analyses were performed: a comparison of the data from all studies irrespective of whether the conditions under which the in vitro study was conducted fully matched those of the in vivo study, and comparison of the data from only those studies in which full harmonization of the experimental conditions existed between the in vitro and in vivo studies. In vitro to in vivo (IVIV) correlation was examined by calculating the ratio of total absorption in vitro/total absorption in vivo, where total absorption was reported as a percent of the applied dose.

Examination of the IVIV ratios for all 92 data sets showed a definite trend for the observed values to follow the line of perfect 1:1 correlation (**Fig. 2**). The average IVIV BA ratio for all 92 data sets was 1.6; however, variability was relatively large, and IVIV BA ratios ranged from 0.18 to 19.7. A substantial improvement in correlation was found in the subset of data from in vitro studies in which the experimental conditions matched those used in vivo in all critical aspects. Eleven data-sets were identified in which the in vitro protocol was fully harmonized with the in vivo protocol (**Fig. 3**). The average IVIV BA ratio for the group now approached 1 (0.96), and the ratio for any individual data set differed from exact correlation (ie, a ratio of 1.0) by less than twofold (the ratios ranged from 0.58 to 1.28).

This analysis effectively demonstrated that absorption data obtained from the excised human skin IVPT model can closely match those obtained in living humans if the experimental conditions match those found in vivo. The two factors leading to exclusion of most of the original 92 data sets were the use of skin from different body sites and different formulations of the compound under study. The latter factor (discrimination of the BA from different formulations) is of special significance, as it is most relevant to the use of the model for BE testing.

In Vitro/In Vivo Correlation: Clinical Studies

Studies that support the use of the excised human skin IVPT model specifically for establishing the BE of topical drug products have been presented by

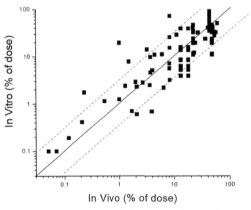

Fig. 2. IVIV ratios of total absorption for 92 data sets plotted on a log-log scale. Ratios ranged from 0.18 to 19.7, with an overall mean of 1.6. Solid line denotes ideal 1:1 correlation, and dashed lines denote ± threefold difference from ideal. (*From* Lehman PA, Raney SG, Franz TJ. Percutaneous absorption in man: in vitro-in vivo correlation. Skin Pharmacol Physiol 2011;24(4):224-30; with permission.)

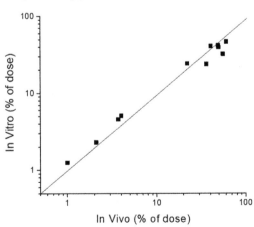

Fig. 3. IVIV ratios of total absorption for 11 fully harmonized data sets plotted on a log-log scale. IVIV ratios ranged from 0.58 to 1.28, with an overall mean of 0.96. Solid line denotes ideal 1:1 correlation. (*From* Lehman PA, Raney SG, Franz TJ. Percutaneous absorption in man: in vitro-in vivo correlation. Skin Pharmacol Physiol 2011;24(4):224-30; with permission.)

Franz and colleagues.[38] Seven prospective generic topical drug products (5 glucocorticoid creams and ointments and 2 tretinoin gels) were evaluated during their preclinical development. Absorption of the active pharmaceutical ingredient (API) was compared side by side to the reference products in the excised human skin IVPT model. All of the test products were later evaluated clinically (by a comparative clinical endpoint study or an in vivo vasoconstrictor assay) and shown to be BE to their respective reference products, thus, affording a unique opportunity to test and demonstrate the validity of the IVPT model to assess BE for topically applied drugs.

In agreement with the clinical data, the IVPT results showed that the BA of the test products were a remarkably close match to that of the reference products. Both tretinoin absorption studies were run as simulated BE studies and a sufficient number of replicate skin sections were included to calculate confidence intervals (Table 1). All parameters fell within the traditional BE limits (0.80–1.25) except for the maximum absorption rate of the 0.025% gel product, which fell slightly outside the upper bound of 1.25.

The 5 glucocorticoid studies were not designed as simulated BE studies but instead as screening studies in which only nine skin sections per product were evaluated. Several test formulations of each drug were initially compared to several lots of the reference products with the objective of selecting the best match (targeting a test/reference approximately 1.0) to move into a pivotal vasoconstrictor study. Of the 5 test formulations selected for clinical study, mometasone furoate

was the only one in which the test/reference ratio (0.63) was not close to 1 (Table 2).

Yet, by vasoconstrictor assay, it and the other four glucocorticoids were found to be bioequivalent to the reference products and subsequently approved. This one instance of an apparent lack of agreement between IVPT and vasoconstrictor assay was determined not to be caused by a shortcoming in the IVPT model but potentially because of a greater discrimination sensitivity of the IVPT relative to the vasoconstrictor assay. An example of this is seen in Table 2, where alclometasone cream and ointment appear approximately equipotent by vasoconstrictor assay, yet differ by more than 15-fold in absorption when assessed by an IVPT.

In another study by Shin and colleagues, the effect of heat on nicotine BA was evaluated following topical application of nicotine transdermal delivery systems (TDS) both in vitro (using IVPT) and in vivo (human serum sampling). The study designs used for both IVPT and in vivo PK study were harmonized and included application of 1 hour transient heat after TDS application. An in vitro–in vivo correlation (IVIVC) was established for nicotine BA, and the result of this work showed that a well-designed and well-controlled IVPT study can be used to assess the relative heat effect on nicotine BA from the TDS products and can be predictive of the heat effect that was observed in vivo.[39]

In summary, IVPT is widely regarded as a valid method by which to quantify the absorption of chemicals into and through human skin, and this acceptance can be justified on the basis of good in vitro/in vivo correlation. Validation of IVPT data has also been specifically extended into the

---

Table 1
Comparison of primary in vitro endpoints for two strengths of generic tretinoin gels (test) versus the reference products.

	Test	Reference	Test/Reference	90% CI
0.01% gel				
Total absorbed	3.00	2.97	1.02	0.97–1.07
J_{max}	0.55	0.57	1.04	0.93–1.15
T_{max}	3.60	3.57	1.04	0.92–1.16
0.025% gel				
Total absorbed	3.49	3.47	1.03	0.95–1.10
J_{max}	0.91	0.88	1.11	0.95–1.28
T_{max}	3.66	3.72	0.98	0.97–1.00

Total absorbed = ng/cm²/48 h; J_{max} = maximum rate of absorption, ng/cm²/h; T_{max} = time of maximum rate of absorption, minutes.
  90% confidence interval (CI) is calculated on the ratio of the means of natural log transformed data.
  Test and reference values represent natural log transformed means.
  Data from Franz TJ, Lehman PA, Raney SG. Use of excised human skin to assess the bioequivalence of topical products. Skin Pharmacol Physiol 2009;22(5):276-86.

Table 2
Comparison of data obtained by the in vitro permeation test versus the in vivo vasoconstrictor assay on five generic glucocorticoid (test) products versus the corresponding reference (ref) products

	In Vitro Absorption (ng/cm^2/ 48 h)			In Vivo VC Assay (Negative AUEC$_{0-24 h}$)		
	Test	Ref	Test/Ref	Test	Ref	Test/Ref
Alclometasone cream	4.52	4.39	1.03	18.5	16.8	1.10
Alclometasone ointment	66.95	70.0	0.96	16.0	17.4	0.92
Halobetasol cream	110.4	96.9	1.14	33.1	30.7	1.08
Halobetasol ointment	246.7	256.3	0.96	28.6	28.5	1.00
Mometasone ointment	213.4	338.7	0.63	13.7	12.3	1.11

Listed numbers are mean values.
Data from Franz TJ, Lehman PA, Raney SG. Use of excised human skin to assess the bioequivalence of topical products. Skin Pharmacol Physiol 2009;22(5):276-86.

sphere of BE, where it has been shown that results obtained in the IVPT model are in agreement with those obtained from the clinical studies that were used as the basis for approval of 7 generic drug products. The IVPT model can provide relevant and accurate results with good IVIVC, and provides information regarding the variability in human skin permeation that is representative of the in vivo population of individuals from whom the skin was acquired. Also, it can be reproducible and discriminating. To facilitate its utility in the context of topical BE assessment, the procedures for the conduct of these studies have been increasingly standardized internationally by several expert groups. Commensurate with the power and utility of this method, validated IVPT studies are required to be performed and included within EMA regulatory submissions for all transdermal products.[24] Independently, in vitro (IVRT or IVPT) studies conducted for the purpose of demonstrating BE are required under 21 CFR Part 320 to be reported within ANDA submissions.[40] Also, the FDA recommends an IVPT study to support a demonstration of BE for numerous topical products.[28]

IN VIVO CUTANEOUS (EPIDERMAL) PHARMACOKINETICS

As previously noted, the BA or BE of systemically acting drug products such as an acetaminophen tablet is typically evaluated using PK studies.[41] For a dermal product, however, evaluating the cutaneous PK and quantifying the rate and extent to which drug becomes available in a solid tissue such as the skin has been challenging. Historically, there has been a lot of interest in developing techniques to evaluate the rate and extent of a drug's BA in the topmost layer of the skin, the epidermis.

The stratum corneum (SC), which is composed of the keratinized remains of rapidly dividing epidermal cells bound together by a lipid matrix, is the outer most layer of the epidermis and is the area of the skin that is visible and accessible externally.

Historically, spectroscopy-based techniques such as attenuated total reflectance Fourier transform infrared spectroscopy (ATR-FTIR) have been utilized for the quantification of drugs and to monitor changes in the structure of the SC barrier following the application of locally applied dermal products, either in vitro or following SC removal by tape stripping (TS).[42] Raman spectroscopy-based techniques were largely used for the evaluation of SC thickness.[43] However, recent advances in noninvasive imaging technology suggest that it may be feasible to use Raman based imaging techniques such as simulated Raman scattering (SRS) microscopy as a label-free, nondestructive tool to monitor the permeation of drugs across the different layers of the skin following topical application of dermal drug products.[44] Saar and colleagues illustrated that differences in the rate of permeation of a drug across the intercellular pathway in the SC (compared with the follicular pathway) could be directly observed using SRS, in addition to observing the metamorphosis of the formulation, including precipitation of the drug crystals and permeation of cosolvents.[45]

In 2013, Mateus and colleagues used Confocal Raman Spectroscopy (CRS) to evaluate drug disposition in the skin following topical application of ibuprofen solutions in vivo. Saturated solutions of ibuprofen in propylene glycol (PG) and PG: water (50:50, 75:25 v/v) solutions were simultaneously applied to 5 healthy subjects for 30 minutes. The semi-quantitative assessment from the study indicated that the permeation profiles of ibuprofen across the skin were comparable to previously published TS data.[46] The observed differences in the permeation of ibuprofen from the 3 formulations suggest that it may be feasible to use Raman spectroscopy-based techniques to assess similarities and differences in drug distribution and to evaluate the BA of a drug from a topically applied drug product.

A practical matter impacting the utilization of such technology for dermal drug development is that a potential limitation to the quantification of drugs (or other compounds of interest) in the skin is the signal interference from the skin itself. Another potentially significant limitation is the increasing attenuation of the signal at deeper levels beneath the surface of the skin, potentially impacting the quantitative or semiquantitative measurement of a drug in the deeper epidermis. There are also technical challenges related to how rapidly measurements can be conducted, how compatible specific technologies may be with different APIs, how data analysis can be automated, and how the models can be validated to be sensitive and discriminatory so that they can be used to support product development and regulatory assessments.

Under the Generic Drug User Fee Amendments (GDUFA) science and research program orchestrated by the FDA's Office of Generic Drugs,[47] CRS-based methods are being developed for the noninvasive evaluation of epidermal PK (University of Bath (Grant# 1U01FD006533) and Massachusetts General Hospital/Harvard Medical School (Grant# 1U01FD006698)). Simultaneously, other research groups are developing automated image analysis tools to evaluate drug distribution in the skin; Jeong and colleagues evaluated the uptake of two drugs (minocycline and tazarotene) within human facial skin using a selective visualization method to monitor and quantify local drug distributions within the skin. Specifically, fluorescence lifetime imaging microscopy (FLIM) was used for the study since both molecules have fluorescence lifetimes that are distinct from the skin's autofluorescence. The publication suggests that the approach to data analysis can be generalized, and that integrating the analysis technique with real time or portable instruments will allow rapid assessment of drug distribution in vivo.[48]

In summary, techniques used to evaluate epidermal PK have advanced substantially over the last 25 years. Although TS-based methodologies have been used previously to quantify and compare the BA of topically applied drugs in the SC, more recent advances suggest that it is feasible to use noninvasive Raman spectroscopy-based techniques to monitor the cutaneous PK and drug distribution in the epidermis following topical application on the skin. Nonetheless, there are current challenges related to the use of these spectroscopic methods for monitoring many topical dermatologic drugs (because many of these drugs may not have an unique Raman spectra) and challenges related to the analysis of relatively large amounts of data with substantially greater spatiotemporal resolution compared to data generated with traditional approaches by which BA/BE are currently being evaluated.

IN VIVO CUTANEOUS (DERMAL) PHARMACOKINETICS

A comparison of in vivo dermal PK for topically applied drug products using dermal microdialysis (dMD) and dermal open flow microperfusion (dOFM) is being investigated to use these methodologies for a BE study as an alternative to a comparative clinical endpoint BE study. Both dMD and dOFM are similar in that both use a thin, hollow tube (or, in the case of dOFM, an open metal mesh[49]), referred to as probe that is inserted below the skin surface, into the dermis, and perfused with a physiologic solution so that drug can be collected in the perfusate from the surrounding tissue.[17,49,50]

In dMD, the probe has a polymeric, porous semipermeable membrane that is often made from material that is the same as or similar to kidney dialysis filters. The porous membrane allows the exchange of analytes (e.g., a drug) between the continuously perfused isotonic fluid and the dermal interstitial fluid (ISF) via passive diffusion across the dialysis membrane. Thus, only drugs that are unbound and soluble in the ISF can be measured using dMD probes, and the collected dialysate is free of proteins or other large molecules and can typically be analyzed without any sample preparation (cleaning).[51]

In dOFM, the membrane is a fenestrated metal mesh, and it uses a push/pull mechanism to collect diluted ISF containing the analyte (drug) of interest (including both bound and unbound drugs).[52] Thus, theoretically, drugs can be quantified using the dOFM technique irrespective of their protein binding characteristics or their lipophilicity; however, the samples collected using this technique often require processing to clean up the sample prior to quantitative analysis.[53]

In both dMD and dOFM, the insertion of the probe is associated with mild discomfort that can be reduced or eliminated by the use of local analgesia (eg, the application of ice packs). However, the probe insertion produces a localized trauma that leads to histamine release and subsequent local hyperemia and edema. For this reason, a period of time (eg, 60–90 minutes or more) is typically needed for the tissue reaction to subside and for physiologic re-equilibration, prior to starting an experiment.[51]

A comprehensive discussion of the procedures related to dMD studies can be found in the article by Holmgaard and colleagues[51] and of the procedures related to dOFM in articles by Bodenlenz and colleagues[53,54] As discussed by Holmgaard and colleagues, the designs of dMD probes differ in size, shape, and material and are selected based on the intended site of implantation.[51] Linear probes are usually thinner and more flexible and cause less tissue disruption during insertion; therefore, they are the most widely used probes for dMD. In most cases, a guide cannula is used to insert the dialysis probe into the middermis (ideally a depth of 0.6–1.0 mm) horizontal to the skin surface, typically on the ventral forearm or the thigh. The precise depth within the skin can be determined by ultrasound, and, with practice, consistent placement at approximately the same depth is achievable. Once the cannula is withdrawn, the probe is fixed in place, and one end is connected to a fluid delivery pump and the other end to a collection system. Isotonic saline or another physiologic solution (such as Ringer solution) is pumped through the probe, generally at a low flow rate (0.9–1.5 µL/min) to allow sufficient time for the drug to diffuse from the ISF to the perfusion solution. Nevertheless, a total equilibrium between the 2 phases is not completely achieved, and, to determine the drug concentration in the surrounding tissue fluid, a recovery rate or extraction efficacy is routinely calculated, defined as the ratio of drug concentration in the dialysate to that in the surrounding tissue fluid. A recovery rate can be obtained from several different procedures and depends on the experimental conditions.[54,55] As an example, in a study by Kuzma and colleagues in Yucatan mini pigs, the BA of metronidazole from metronidazole topical gel and a cream product was evaluated.[56] In this study, deuterated (D3)-metronidazole was used as an internal standard to calibrate the dMD method, and it was added to the physiologic buffer that was perfused through dMD probes. The concentration of D3-metronidazole was measured in the dialysate samples, and a correction factor (defined as the relative loss of the D3-metronidazole compared with the concentration in the perfusate) was used to monitor probe performance through the duration of the study and to estimate the actual concentration of metronidazole in dermal ISF. That being said, although using a recovery rate or correction factor can be critically important in some research areas, its use for BE may not be essential, as the test/reference ratio in the dialysate (the relative amounts rather than the absolute amounts) can be the basis for a statistical comparison of data obtained for the test and reference products.

Because of the hydrophilic nature of the perfusion fluid, adequate recovery of lipophilic drugs can be challenging. The perfusate can be modified by the inclusion of serum albumin or other additives such as Intralipid, Encapsin, or cyclodextrins to improve recovery. However, in a study in which estradiol absorption from a commercial TDS was examined, detectable drug levels were found in only 8 of 10 in vitro experiments in spite of the addition of 7% serum albumin to the perfusion fluid.[57] Likewise, the measurement of glucocorticoid absorption in humans following topical application has only been reported with 4% clobetasol propionate in alcohol using Intralipid in the perfusate, but not with any commercial products at the most common 0.05% clobetasol propionate product strength.[58]

Clinical Correlation

Substantial work has been done in humans to demonstrate the feasibility of dMD and dOFM for measuring the cutaneous BA of drugs following topical application. Several of these studies have special relevance to BA and BE, because they involve a direct comparison of the rate and extent of topically applied drug absorption from different vehicles, and confirm the ability of dMD to accurately confirm a comparable dermal PK for products having equal BA and sensitively discriminate differences in the dermal PK between products with inequivalent BA. For example, Kreilgaard and colleagues used dMD to compare the absorption of 5% lidocaine from a commercial product to that of a laboratory-made microemulsion formulation and found greater absorption from the microemulsion vehicle.[59] Over the 4-hour collection period, the average areas under the curve (AUCs) were 2900 plus or minus 2690 versus 867 plus or minus 488 mg/L for the microemulsion and commercial product, respectively. The lag time was also found to be shorter for the microemulsion compared with the commercial product, 87 versus 110 minutes, respectively ($P<.02$). A second part of the study compared the PK results obtained by dMD with a pharmacodynamic (PD) response, pain reduction. Both products diminished the pain elicited by a standardized stimulus compared with a placebo microemulsion, but the PD test could not distinguish between the 2 active products, illustrating the greater sensitivity of dermal

Table 3
Comparison of lidocaine permeation from a cream and ointment formulation determined by dermal microdialysis

	AUC[a] (ng/mL/min)	C_{max}[a] (ng/mL)	Lag Time[b] (min)
Cream			
Mean	15,983	112	26.0
CV (%)	41	41	18
Ointment			
Mean	3309	27.5	45.6
CV (%)	42	41	27
t-test (P value)	0.018	0.03	0.06

[a] Geometric mean.
[b] Time at which drug level exceeded the lower limit of quantitation.
   Adapted from Benfeldt E, Hansen SH, Volund A, Menne T, Shah VP. Bioequivalence of topical formulations in humans: evaluation by dermal microdialysis sampling and the dermatopharmacokinetic method. J Invest Dermatol 2007;127(1):170-8; with permission.

PK endpoints monitored by dMD relative to the PD endpoints.

Benfeldt and colleagues also evaluated the relative BA of lidocaine.[60] Two commercial 5% products (cream and ointment) were applied at different times to the ventral forearms of 8 subjects. Each was applied to 2 separate sites, and drug permeation was assessed using 2 dialysis probes per site. Analysis of the AUC over the 5-hour collection period showed an almost fivefold greater absorption from the cream product (**Table 3**). Of note, no statistically significant difference was seen between the results obtained from the 4 separate probes. In analyzing total variance, 19% was associated with differences between probes, 20% was caused by a difference between the 2 dosing sites, and 61% was caused by intersubject variability.

Tettey-Amlalo and colleagues examined the use of dMD for BE by measuring ketoprofen permeation in 18 subjects.[61] A single commercial 2.5% gel product was applied to 4 separate forearm sites and the dialysate collected over a 5-hour period from one probe per site. The experimental design allowed 2 sites each to be assigned as mock test and reference sites and, because 4 sites were available, 3 different randomization schemes could be used (TTRR/RRTT, TRTR/RTRT, TRRT/RTTR) to assess the BE of the test and reference products. Intrasubject variability for probes averaged approximately 10%, whereas intersubject variability for each probe averaged approximately 68%. Although the BE assessment for all 3 randomization schemes found the confidence interval for the test/reference ratio of log transformed data to fall within 0.80 and 1.25, 1 of the 3 sequences was found to lack the 90% power (**Table 4**). It was suggested that this may have been caused by regional variation within the forearm itself, which has been reported before,[62] because the aberrant sequence was the one comparing the most proximal and distal sites

Table 4
Comparison of ketoprofen permeation from a single 2.5% gel randomly assigned as both test and reference to 4 adjacent sites on the forearm

Sequence	AUC_{0-5} (ng/mL/h)		Statistical Analysis	
	Test[a]	Reference[a]	90% CI[b]	Power of ANOVA (%)
TTRR/RRTT	155.5 ± 98.9	150.0 ± 107.3	0.97–1.15	92.88
TRTR/RTRT	152.0 ± 99.2	153.5 ± 103.9	0.90–1.09	95.95
TRRT/RTTR	139.9 ± 87.3	165.6 ± 116.7	0.80–0.94	53.99

[a] mean ± SD.
[b] 90% confidence interval (CI) calculated on the ratio of the means (test/reference) using log transformed data.
   Adapted from Tettey-Amlalo RN, Kanfer I, Skinner MF, Benfeldt E, Verbeeck RK. Application of dermal microdialysis for the evaluation of bioequivalence of a ketoprofen topical gel. Eur J Pharm Sci 2009;36(2–3):219-25; with permission.

(both having low AUCs) with the 2 middle sites (both having high AUCs).

Another study having a similar objective of specifically using dMD for evaluating the BE of various drug products was that of Garcia Ortiz and colleagues[63] Metronidazole permeation from 3 commercial products, approved as being BE in Europe, was measured concurrently in 14 subjects. Each product was randomly assigned to 1 of 3 adjacent sites on the ventral forearm, and 3 probes were inserted per site. Although no statistically significant differences in AUC ($P>.05$) were found following a 5-hour collection period, and there was high intersubject variability (116%–223%), and none of the products met traditional criteria for BE (the 90% CI calculated for the ratio of the means using log transformed data fell outside the bound of 0.80–1.25 for all comparisons of the 3 products to each other). It was estimated that 34 subjects would have been needed to attain sufficient statistical power for this analysis.

Although the aforementioned studies demonstrate the potential of dermal PK sampling techniques to assess the BA/BE of topical dermatologic products, 1 major limitation that existed in all of those studies had been the short duration of the study (eg, 4–6 hours), which may not be sufficient to adequately capture the dermal PK profile of topically applied drugs. Perhaps the most compelling evidence supporting the use of dermal PK to evaluate topical BE in human subjects comes from the work of Bodenlenz and colleagues, who compared the topical BA of acyclovir from test and reference products.[54] Among the notable advancements of their approach was the use of small portable pumps that allowed the subjects in the study sufficient mobility that the dermal PK could be monitored continuously for 34 hours. In addition, the investigators used dOFM probes and introduced several procedural controls into the study design, including the use of duplicate sets of probes and templates to stabilize anatomic flexion of the upper leg (thigh), where the probes were inserted, to enhance the precision of the results and the discrimination sensitivity of the methodology. Using traditional BE PK endpoints of C_{max} and AUC, and traditional BE limits of 80% to 125%, the investigators compared the reference product to itself as a positive control for BE, and compared the reference product to a test product as a negative control for BE. The positive control products were accurately shown to be bioequivalent, while the negative control products were discriminated as not being bioequivalent, both in the same population of the 20 subjects.

A noteworthy and unique advantage of dMD and dOFM over other cutaneous PK-based techniques is their ability to be used in diseased skin; this not only allows for measuring drug concentrations at or near the site(s) of action in the skin, but also for monitoring the intradermal biochemistry in patient populations to establish PK/PD relationships. In a pilot study by Quist and colleagues, 6 patients with chronic plaque psoriasis received methotrexate either orally or through subcutaneous injection and the drug concentration in dermal ISF was measured using dMD in psoriasis plaque and non-lesional skin, and in plasma using blood sampling for 10 hours.[64] Methotrexate levels and $AUC_{0-10\ h}$ were reported to be higher in lesional than nonlesional psoriatic skin and also much lower than those in the blood samples. In another study, 12 patients with moderate atopic dermatitis (AD) received topical treatment on either arm with tacrolimus topical ointment, 0.1% or a lotion containing 12% ω-6 fatty acids (polyunsaturated fatty acids; PUFA) twice daily for 5 consecutive days.[65] On day 6, dMD sampling was performed, and dialysate samples were collected at 30-minute intervals for 8 hours from 4 defined skin areas: lesional, nonlesional, and topically treated skin (treated with either tacrolimus or PUFA). Markers of oxidative stress (F2-isoprostanes; 5- and 8-prostaglandin F2α) and inflammation (9α,11α-prostaglandin F2α; and prostaglandin E2) were quantified. The results of this dMD study demonstrated that treatment with tacrolimus compared with PUFA appears to suppress eicosanoids more efficiently in AD skin, and the levels of eicosanoids were increased in clinically lesional skin compared with nonlesional AD skin. Bodenlenz and colleagues also investigated the PK of a highly lipophilic antipsoriatic drug using dOFM.[66] In that study, 12 patients received Dermovate (clobetasol propionate) topical cream, 0.05% once daily on small lesional and nonlesional skin test sites for 14 consecutive days. On days 1 and 14, dermal ISF was sampled by dOFM continuously from baseline to 24 hours after the dose while the cream remained on the skin and a nonocclusive dressing was used to protect the test sites. On day 1, quantifiable drug concentrations in the dermal ISF of nonlesional skin was obtained at approximately 10 hours after the dose, and maximum concentrations were observed at 18 hours after the dose (mean C_{max} 0.61 ng/mL). In lesional skin, the drug levels steadily increased on day 1 but did not reach the lower limit of quantitation (LLOQ) during the entire 24-hour sampling period in most subjects (mean C_{max} 0.19 ng/mL). On day 14, the C_{max} (mean C_{max} 1.00 ng/mL) was reached at 10 hours in nonlesional skin, while in lesional skin, the clobetasol propionate levels were already quantifiable at baseline (before the dose), and moderately increased after dosing to reach C_{max} at 18 h (mean C_{max} 0.68 ng/mL). Overall, the authors concluded that the thickened psoriatic stratum corneum can decrease the skin permeation rate for lipophilic topical drugs like clobetasol propionate.

In summary, dermal PK techniques such as dMD and dOFM can directly monitor the dynamic concentrations of a drug in the dermis, which, for most dermatologic drugs, is at or near their site of action. Several studies have demonstrated the ability of these dermal PK techniques to monitor the permeation of several topically applied drugs with good sensitivity to distinguish differences in a drug's BA when applied in different vehicles. Based on the experimental variability observed in these studies, it is reasonable to expect that a well-controlled dMD or dOFM study would often have sufficient power to establish BE with a few dozen subjects. The results from 1 study on lidocaine absorption suggested that current traditional statistical requirements could be met with as few as 18 subjects, whereas another study with metronidazole estimated that 34 subjects would be needed. Similarly, the results from the dOFM clinical study with acyclovir demonstrated that 19 subjects would have been sufficient to have satisfied traditional BE criteria. Distinct limitations of dMD include potential difficulties in detecting drugs that are highly lipophilic or protein bound, and possibly the length of time that subjects can be comfortably immobilized with dialysis probes in place (if the dMD probes are not used with portable pumps). Further research with dOFM and dMD is certainly warranted, particularly to evaluate the utility of these techniques to monitor the dermal PK of drugs that are more lipophilic and protein bound than acyclovir.

SUMMARY

The practical assessment of BE for each drug product is not a one-dimensional issue, but rather, it routinely involves characterizing a multidimensional topography of product attributes and behavior that together define product performance in each case. As understanding of the physiochemical and structural complexity of semisolid drug products has evolved, it has become increasingly clear that the components, composition, and arrangement of matter in topical dermatologic products can be critical to their clinical performance.[67,68] Thus, it is important to consider such molecular and macromolecular qualities in the design of bioequivalent drug products, characterizing them as rigorously as possible. This might include matching characteristics like texture, rheology, specific gravity, phase state(s), particle size and distribution of the drug substance(s), globule size and distribution, polymorphic forms, pH, and other potentially critical physicochemical and structural characteristics, as relevant to a product. It may not always be possible to identify and perfectly match the arrangement of matter between a test and reference topical dermatologic drug product (or even between manufacturing batches of a test or reference product), and so appropriate in vitro and/or in vivo tests of product performance serve an important role as part of a multicomponent risk-based assessment of BE. As discussed in this work, it is now feasible for evidence from in vitro and/or in vivo cutaneous PK approaches to support a demonstration of BE.

A single approach alone may not always be sufficient to demonstrate BE, but the collective weight of evidence from orthogonal methods can be highly effective in affirming BE. The rational selection of such test methods, used in combination with rigorous physicochemical and structural characterization of the drug product, is particularly valuable for the evaluation of multidimensional aspects of product quality and performance that can collectively support a demonstration of BE. Such approaches, and in particular, cutaneous PK approaches to compare BA and/or BE for topical dermatologic drug products, will likely provide an efficient path forward for developers and regulators of topical semisolid generic drug products, where no viable path had previously existed, and to provide patients with access to generic topical medications whose qualities and performance have been evaluated and matched to those of the reference product more comprehensively than ever before.

CLINICS CARE POINTS

- Cutaneous pharmacokinetics based bioequivalence approaches ensure that topical generic products are safe and effective with the same rate and extent of drug bioavailability.

- Topical generic products approved using in vitro cutaneous pharmacokinetics based bioequivalence approaches additionally have the same look and feel as the brand name product.

DISCLOSURE

The information and opinions expressed in this article reflect the views of the authors and do not necessarily reflect the views or policies of the FDA or any other organizations with which the authors are affiliated.

REFERENCES

1. Title 21 of the U.S. Code of Federal Regulations, Part 320. Available at: http://www.accessdata.fda.gov/scripts/cdrh/cfdocs/cfcfr/CFRSearch.cfm?CFRPart=320. Accessed January 4, 2022.
2. Midha KK, McKay G. Bioequivalence; its history, practice, and future. AAPS J 2009;11(4):664–70.
3. The Drug Price Competition and Patent Term Restoration Act of 1984 (Public Law 98-417; 98th Congress). September 24, 1984. Available at. https://www.gpo.gov/fdsys/pkg/STATUTE-98/pdf/STATUTE-98-Pg1585.pdf. Accessed January 4, 2022.
4. The Medicare Prescription Drug, Improvement and Modernization Act of 2003 (Public Law 108-173; 108th Congress). 2003. Available at: https://www.gpo.gov/fdsys/pkg/PLAW-108publ173/pdf/PLAW-108publ173.pdf. Accessed January 4, 2022.
5. Section 320.24 (21 CFR § 320.24: Types of evidence to measure bioavailability or establish bioequivalence) of Title 21 of the U.S. Code of Federal Regulations. Available at. https://www.gpo.gov/fdsys/granule/CFR-2012-title21-vol5/CFR-2012-title21-vol5-sec320-24. Accessed January 4, 2022.
6. FDA Guidance for Industry: Topical Dermatologic Corticosteroids: In Vivo Bioequivalence. 1995. Available at: http://www.fda.gov/downloads/Drugs/GuidanceComplianceRegulatoryInformation/Guidances/ucm070234.pdf. Accessed January 4, 2022.
7. Skelly J, Shah V, Maibach H, et al. FDA and AAPS report of the workshop on principles and practices of in vitro percutaneous penetration studies: relevance to bioavailability and bioequivalence. Pharm Res 1987;4:265–7.
8. Pershing LK, Silver BS, Krueger GG, et al. Feasibility of measuring the bioavailability of topical betamethasone dipropionate in commercial formulations using drug content in skin and a skin blanching bioassay. Pharm Res 1992;9(1):45–51.
9. Pershing L, Lambert L, Shah V, et al. Variability and correlation of chromameter and tape-stripping methods with the visual skin blanching assay in the quantitative assessment of topical 0.05% betamethasone dipropionate bioavailability in humans. Int J Pharm 1992;86(2–3):201–10.
10. Shah VP, Behl CR, Flynn GL, et al. Principles and criteria in the development and optimization of topical therapeutic products. Pharm Res 1992;9(8):1107–11.
11. Shah V, Elkins J, Williams R. In vitro drug release measurement for topical glucocorticoid creams. Pharmacopeial Forum 1993;19:5048–60.
12. FDA Guidance for Industry: Nonsterile Semisolid Dosage Forms, Scale-up and Post-Approval Changes: Chemistry, Manufacturing, and Controls; In Vitro Release Testing and In Vivo Bioequivalence Documentation. 1997. Available at: http://www.fda.gov/downloads/Drugs/GuidanceComplianceRegulatoryInformation/Guidances/UCM070930.pdf. Accessed January 4, 2022.
13. Shah VP, Flynn GL, Yacobi A, et al. Bioequivalence of topical dermatological dosage forms–methods of evaluation of bioequivalence. Pharm Res 1998;15(2):167–71.
14. Flynn GL, Shah VP, Tenjarla SN, et al. Assessment of value and applications of in vitro testing of topical dermatological drug products. Pharm Res 1999;16(9):1325–30.
15. Pershing LK, Bakhtian S, Poncelet CE, et al. Comparison of skin stripping, in vitro release, and skin blanching response methods to measure dose response and similarity of triamcinolone acetonide cream strengths from two manufactured sources. J Pharm Sci 2002;91(5):1312–23.
16. Pershing LK, Nelson JL, Corlett JL, et al. Assessment of dermatopharmacokinetic approach in the bioequivalence determination of topical tretinoin gel products. J Am Acad Dermatol 2003;48(5):740–51.
17. Chaurasia CS, Muller M, Bashaw ED, et al. AAPS-FDA workshop white paper: microdialysis principles, application and regulatory perspectives. Pharm Res 2007;24(5):1014–25.
18. Herkenne C, Alberti I, Naik A, et al. In vivo methods for the assessment of topical drug bioavailability. Pharm Res 2008;25(1):87–103.
19. N'Dri-Stempfer B, Navidi WC, Guy RH, et al. Optimizing metrics for the assessment of bioequivalence between topical drug products. Pharm Res 2008;25(7):1621–30.
20. N'Dri-Stempfer B, Navidi WC, Guy RH, et al. Improved bioequivalence assessment of topical dermatological drug products using dermatopharmacokinetics. Pharm Res 2009;26(2):316–28.
21. Raney SG, Franz TJ, Lehman PA, et al. Pharmacokinetics-based approaches for bioequivalence evaluation of topical dermatological drug products. Clin Pharmacokinet 2015;54(11):1095–106.
22. Organisation for Economic Cooperation and Development. OECD guideline for testing of chemicals No. 428: skin absorption: in vitro methods. Paris (France): OECD; 2004. p. 1–8.
23. Organisation for Economic Cooperation and Development. OECD series on testing and assessment

No. 28: guidance document for the conduct of skin absorption studies: OECD. 2004:1-31.

24. EMA/CHMP/QWP/608924/2014, guideline on quality of transdermal patches. 2014. Available at: http://www.ema.europa.eu/docs/en_GB/document_library/Scientific_guideline/2014/12/WC500179071.pdf. Accessed January 4, 2022.

25. EPA (US Environmental Protection Agency). Reregistration eligibility decision (RED) for permethrin. Case No. 2510. U.S. EPA 738-R-09-306. Washington (DC): Office of Prevention, Pesticides, and Toxic Substances; 2009.

26. Reifenrath WG, Ross JH, Driver JH. Experimental methods for determining permethrin dermal absorption. J Toxicol Environ Health A 2011;74(5):325-35.

27. Ross JH, Reifenrath WG, Driver JH. Estimation of the percutaneous absorption of permethrin in humans using the parallelogram method. J Toxicol Environ Health A 2011;74(6):351-63.

28. U.S. FDA. Product-specific guidances for generic drug development. Available at: https://www.fda.gov/drugs/guidances-drugs/product-specific-guidances-generic-drug-development. Accessed January 4, 2022.

29. Franz TJ, Lehman PA, Raney SG. The cadaver skin absorption model and the drug development process. Pharmacopeial Forum 2008;34:1349-56.

30. Howes D, Guy R, Hadgraft J, et al. Methods for assessing percutaneous absorption: the report and recommendations of ECVAM workshop 13. Altern Lab Anim 1996;24(1):81-106.

31. Kielhorn J, Melching-Korllmuss S, Mangelsforf I. WHO (World Health Organization). International Programme on Chemical Safety, Environmental Health Ccriteria 235, Dermal Absorption. Geneva (Switzerland): WHO Press; 2005.

32. Basic criteria for the in vitro assessment of dermal absorption of cosmetic ingredients. In: SCCS (Scientific Committee on Consumer Safety). 2010. Available at: http://ec.europa.eu/health/scientific_committees/consumer_safety/docs/sccs_s_002.pdf. Accessed January 4, 2022.

33. Bronaugh RL, Stewart RF. Methods for in vitro percutaneous absorption studies III: hydrophobic compounds. J Pharm Sci 1984;73(9):1255-8.

34. Bronaugh RL, Stewart RF. Methods for in vitro percutaneous absorption studies. VI: Preparation of the barrier layer. J Pharm Sci 1986;75(5):487-91.

35. Scott RC, Ramsey JD. Comparison of the in vivo and in vitro percutaneous absorption of a lipophilic molecule (cypermethrin, a pyrethroid insecticide). J Invest Dermatol 1987;89(2):142-6.

36. Ramsey JD, Woollen BH, Auton TR, et al. The predictive accuracy of in vitro measurements for the dermal absorption of a lipophilic penetrant (fluazifop-butyl) through rat and human skin. Fundam Appl Toxicol 1994;23(2):230-6.

37. Lehman PA, Raney SG, Franz TJ. Percutaneous absorption in man: in vitro-in vivo correlation. Skin Pharmacol Physiol 2011;24(4):224-30.

38. Franz TJ, Lehman PA, Raney SG. Use of excised human skin to assess the bioequivalence of topical products. Skin Pharmacol Physiol 2009;22(5):276-86.

39. Shin SH, Thomas S, Raney SG, et al. In vitro-in vivo correlations for nicotine transdermal delivery systems evaluated by both in vitro skin permeation (IVPT) and in vivo serum pharmacokinetics under the influence of transient heat application. J Control Release 2018;270:76-88.

40. Guidance for industry: submission of summary bioequivalence data for ANDAs. 2011. Available at: http://www.fda.gov/downloads/Drugs/GuidanceComplianceRegulatoryInformation/Guidances/UCM134846.pdf. Accessed January 4, 2022.

41. Guidance for industry: bioequivalence studies with pharmacokinetic endpoints for drugs submitted under an abbreviated new drug application. 2021. Available at: https://www.fda.gov/regulatory-information/search-fda-guidance-documents/bioequivalence-studies-pharmacokinetic-endpoints-drugs-submitted-under-abbreviated-new-drug. Accessed January 4, 2022.

42. Ibrahim SA, Li SK. Chemical enhancer solubility in human stratum corneum lipids and enhancer mechanism of action on stratum corneum lipid domain. Int J Pharm 2010;383(1-2):89-98.

43. Caspers PJ, Lucassen GW, Wolthuis R, et al. In vitro and in vivo Raman spectroscopy of human skin. Biospectroscopy 1998;4(5 Suppl):S31-9.

44. Pena AM, Chen X, Pence IJ, et al. Imaging and quantifying drug delivery in skin - part 2: fluorescence and vibrational spectroscopic imaging methods. Adv Drug Deliv Rev 2020;153:147-68.

45. Saar BG, Contreras-Rojas LR, Xie XS, et al. Imaging drug delivery to skin with stimulated Raman scattering microscopy. Mol Pharm 2011;8(3):969-75.

46. Mateus R, Abdalghafor H, Oliveira G, et al. A new paradigm in dermatopharmacokinetics - confocal Raman spectroscopy. Int J Pharm 2013;444(1-2):106-8.

47. FY2020 GDUFA science and research report. Available at: https://www.fda.gov/drugs/generic-drugs/fy2020-gdufa-science-and-research-report. Accessed January 4, 2022.

48. Jeong S, Greenfield DA, Hermsmeier M, et al. Time-resolved fluorescence microscopy with phasor analysis for visualizing multicomponent topical drug distribution within human skin. Sci Rep 2020;10(1):5360.

49. Bodenlenz M, Hofferer C, Magnes C, et al. Dermal PK/PD of a lipophilic topical drug in psoriatic patients by continuous intradermal membrane-free sampling. Eur J Pharm Biopharm 2012;81(3):635-41.

50. de Lange EC, Ravenstijn PG, Groenendaal D, et al. Toward the prediction of CNS drug-effect profiles in physiological and pathological conditions using microdialysis and mechanism-based pharmacokinetic-pharmacodynamic modeling. AAPS J 2005; 7(3):E532–43.

51. Holmgaard R, Nielsen JB, Benfeldt E. Microdialysis sampling for investigations of bioavailability and bioequivalence of topically administered drugs: current state and future perspectives. Skin Pharmacol Physiol 2010;23(5):225–43.

52. Holmgaard R, Benfeldt E, Nielsen JB, et al. Comparison of open-flow microperfusion and microdialysis methodologies when sampling topically applied fentanyl and benzoic acid in human dermis ex vivo. Pharm Res 2012;29(7):1808–20.

53. Bodenlenz M, Aigner B, Dragatin C, et al. Clinical applicability of dOFM devices for dermal sampling. Skin Res Technol 2013;19(4):474–83.

54. Bodenlenz M, Tiffner KI, Raml R, et al. Open flow microperfusion as a dermal pharmacokinetic approach to evaluate topical bioequivalence. Clin Pharmacokinet 2017;56(1):99.

55. Müller M, Schmid R, Georgopoulos A, et al. Application of microdialysis to clinical pharmacokinetics in humans. Clin Pharmacol Ther 1995;57(4):371–80.

56. Kuzma BA, Senemar S, Ramezanli T, et al. Evaluation of local bioavailability of metronidazole from topical formulations using dermal microdialysis: preliminary study in a Yucatan mini-pig model. Eur J Pharm Sci 2021;159:105741.

57. Müller M, Schmid R, Wagner O, et al. In vivo characterization of transdermal drug transport by microdialysis. J controlled release 1995;37(1–2):49–57.

58. Au WL, Skinner MF, Benfeldt E, et al. Application of dermal microdialysis for the determination of bioavailability of clobetasol propionate applied to the skin of human subjects. Skin Pharmacol Physiol 2012;25(1):17–24.

59. Kreilgaard M, Kemme MJ, Burggraaf J, et al. Influence of a microemulsion vehicle on cutaneous bioequivalence of a lipophilic model drug assessed by microdialysis and pharmacodynamics. Pharm Res 2001;18(5):593–9.

60. Benfeldt E, Hansen SH, Volund A, et al. Bioequivalence of topical formulations in humans: evaluation by dermal microdialysis sampling and the dermatopharmacokinetic method. J Invest Dermatol 2007; 127(1):170–8.

61. Tettey-Amlalo RN, Kanfer I, Skinner MF, et al. Application of dermal microdialysis for the evaluation of bioequivalence of a ketoprofen topical gel. Eur J Pharm Sci 2009;36(2–3):219–25.

62. Lehman PA, Franz TJ. Assessing the bioequivalence of topical retinoid products by pharmacodynamic assay. Skin Pharmacol Physiol 2012;25(5):269–80.

63. Garcia Ortiz P, Hansen SH, Shah VP, et al. Are marketed topical metronidazole creams bioequivalent? Evaluation by in vivo microdialysis sampling and tape stripping methodology. Skin Pharmacol Physiol 2011;24(1):44–53.

64. Quist SR, Quist J, Birkenmaier J, et al. Pharmacokinetic profile of methotrexate in psoriatic skin via the oral or subcutaneous route using dermal microdialysis showing higher methotrexate bioavailability in psoriasis plaques than in non-lesional skin. J Eur Acad Dermatol Venereol 2016;30(9):1537–43.

65. Quist SR, Wiswedel I, Doering I, et al. Effects of topical tacrolimus and polyunsaturated fatty acids on in vivo release of eicosanoids in atopic dermatitis during dermal microdialysis. Acta Derm Venereol 2016;96(7):905–9.

66. Bodenlenz M, Dragatin C, Liebenberger L, et al. Kinetics of Clobetasol-17-Propionate in psoriatic lesional and non-lesional skin assessed by dermal open flow microperfusion with time and space resolution. Pharm Res 2016;33(9):2229–38.

67. Chang RK, Raw A, Lionberger R, et al. Erratum to: generic development of topical dermatologic products: formulation development, process development, and testing of topical dermatologic products. AAPS J 2015;17(6):1522.

68. Chang RK, Raw A, Lionberger R, et al. Generic development of topical dermatologic products, part II: quality by design for topical semisolid products. AAPS J 2013;15(3):674–83.

Measuring What Matters to Patients in Dermatology Drug Development
A Regulatory Perspective

Selena R. Daniels, PharmD, PhD[a],*, Kendall A. Marcus, MD[b],
Robyn Bent, RN, MS[c], Elektra Papadopoulos, MD, MPH[a]

KEYWORDS

- Dermatology • Measurement • Observer-reported outcomes • Patient-centered
- Patient-focused drug development • Patient-reported outcomes • Regulatory
- Clinical outcome assessments

KEY POINTS

- Integrating the patient voice in dermatologic clinical trials provides the opportunity to capture the patient experience, particularly with symptomatic and aesthetic conditions.
- Patients' views of their symptoms and how they may affect their daily lives are instrumental in treatment decisions in dermatology.
- Inclusion of patient-reported and observer-reported outcomes in dermatologic clinical trials can enable regulators to evaluate new dermatologic agents from a patient-centered perspective.

INTRODUCTION

In an effort to make the science of drug development more patient-centered, the patient voice has been increasingly integrated into the drug development and regulatory review process. Incorporating patient perspective into drug development provides unique insight into the patient's experience, needs, and priorities related to their health condition and treatment, as well as context for regulatory decision-making in the evaluation of the benefits and risks of new products.

In dermatology, capturing the patient voice is particularly relevant because the patient's perspective is critical in evaluating treatment outcomes in symptomatic dermatologic conditions, as well as aesthetic procedures.[1,2] One way to capture the patient voice in drug development is by gathering patient and other stakeholder input on what symptoms and impacts matter most to patients with respect to their disease or condition and can also change with treatment and, subsequently, using appropriate clinical outcome assessments to capture the outcomes of interest. To this end, the United States (US) Food and Drug Administration (FDA) has developed guidance for industry to assist stakeholders in collecting comprehensive, representative, and meaningful information from patients and caregivers,[3,4] and additional guidance on patient-focused clinical outcome assessment is in development.[5]

A patient-reported outcome (PRO) is a type of clinical outcome assessment (COA) that can

[a] Division of Clinical Outcome Assessment, Office of Drug Evaluation Science, Center for Drug Evaluation and Research, U.S. Food and Drug Administration, 10903 New Hampshire Avenue, Silver Spring, MD 20903, USA; [b] Division of Dermatology and Dentistry, Office of New Drugs, Center for Drug Evaluation and Research, U.S. Food and Drug Administration, 10903 New Hampshire Avenue, Silver Spring, MD 20903, USA; [c] Patient Focused Drug Development, Office of Center Director, Center for Drug Evaluation and Research, U.S. Food and Drug Administration, 10903 New Hampshire Avenue, Silver Spring, MD 20903, USA
* Corresponding author.
E-mail address: selena.daniels@fda.hhs.gov

Dermatol Clin 40 (2022) 333–337
https://doi.org/10.1016/j.det.2022.03.002
0733-8635/22/Published by Elsevier Inc.

provide a standardized assessment for collecting data directly from patients about the status of a patient's health condition without amendment or interpretation of the patient's response by a clinician or anyone else.[6]

PRO assessments can provide the opportunity to measure what is most important to patients, as well as generate information regarding clinical benefit of a medical product. The US FDA perspective is that clinical benefit means that the intervention produces a positive, clinically meaningful effect on how a patient feels, functions, or survives. Recently, there has been increased use of PRO assessments in dermatology clinical trials, which may be a result of the emphasis on patient-focused drug development. In this article, the authors provide a US regulatory perspective on the use of PROs in dermatologic clinical trials.

CURRENT LANDSCAPE OF DERMATOLOGIC CLINICAL TRIALS

Traditionally, clinician-reported outcome assessments (ClinROs) have been most used to support primary endpoints in dermatology drug development in the absence of suitable markers of disease activity.[1,7] A ClinRO is a type of COA based on a report that comes from a trained health care professional after observation of a patient's health condition.[6] Many cClinRO assessments incorporate different aspects of disease that are combined in various ways into an overall score to make a visual global assessment.[7]

Although it is important for clinicians to examine the effects of treatments for skin diseases in clinical trials, it is as important to include the patient's perspective regarding their experience with their health condition and the treatments under investigation.[7] Use of patient self-report can provide additional valuable outcome data beyond clinician assessment, particularly as some aspects of the patient experience can only be assessed by the patient (eg, symptoms, satisfaction with treatment).

Historically, the use of PRO assessments in dermatology clinical trials has been limited to aesthetic indications and positioned as co-

primary endpoints along with ClinRO assessments. In recent years, PRO assessments are being used more frequently as secondary endpoints in indications of symptomatic dermatologic conditions (eg, psoriasis, atopic dermatitis) as evidenced by inclusion of PRO data in US FDA labeling (**Table 1**).

In instances where patients in the target population are expected to be unable to validly and provide reliably self-report (eg, infants and young children), assessments by a caregiver or other observer based on clearly defined, observable signs have been used in dermatology clinical trials. For example, observable signs of scratching/rubbing, bleeding, or vocalizing responses to itch (eg, "I'm itchy") can be reported using an observer-reported outcome (ObsRO) assessment, a type of COA based on a report of observable signs, events, or behaviors related to a patient's health condition by someone other than the patient or a health professional. Generally, ObsROs are reported by a parent, caregiver, or someone who observes the patient in daily life and are particularly useful for patients who cannot report for themselves.[6] ObsRO assessments are another

Table 1
Examples of dermatologic indications with inclusion of patient-reported outcome data

Condition	Concept	PRO Tool Type
Atopic dermatitis	Itching intensity	Numeric Rating Scale
Interdigital tinea pedis, tinea cruris, tinea corporis	Pruritus symptoms	Pruritus assessment
Plaque psoriasis	Plaque psoriasis symptoms	Signs and symptoms measures[a]
	Itching severity	Numeric Rating Scale
Submental fat	Submental convexity or fullness	Patient-Reported Submental Fat Rating Scale
	Visual and emotional impact of submental fat	6-item survey

[a] Specific measure of psoriasis signs and symptoms vary across drug development programs.

Adapted from FDA. Clinical Outcome Assessment Compendium (COA Compendium), updated June 2021. *Available from*: https://www.fda.gov/media/130138/download [Accessed August 20, 2021b].

Table 2
Examples of dermatologic conditions represented in Food and Drug Administration–led patient-focused drug development and externally led patient-focused drug development meetings

FDA-Led PFDD Meetings	Externally-Led PFDD Meetings
Psoriasis (2016)	Hyperhidrosis (2017)
Alopecia areata (2017)	Pachyonychia congenita (2018)
Vitiligo (2021)	Epidermolysis bullosa (2018)
—	Eczema (2019)

way to incorporate the patient experience in dermatology drug development.

Patient-Focused Drug Development Initiative

To promote patient-focused drug development (PFDD), FDA established the PFDD initiative in 2012 under the fifth authorization of the Prescription Drug User Fee Act (PDUFA V) to methodically obtain patient input on specific health conditions and associated treatments in the format of a meeting. PFDD meetings are distinct from FDA public meetings, as they are designed to engage patients and elicit their perspectives on what is most important to patients in relation to the symptoms of their condition and how they may affect their daily lives, as well as their current approaches to treatment. FDA-led PFDD meetings have provided a forum to key stakeholders, which include FDA, patient advocacy groups, researchers, drug developers, health care providers, and others, to hear the patient's voice. These meetings have been informative and give insight on patients' specific experiences that matter most to them; their perspectives on meaningful treatment benefits; and their interest to be engaged in the drug development process. By understanding patient's concerns, we are better able to include endpoints that are meaningful to patients and prescribers.

To date FDA has conducted 30 disease-specific PFDD meetings, including dermatologic areas (**Table 2**). Patient organizations have also led their own PFDD meetings to help expand the benefits of FDA's PFDD initiative and to generate public input on other disease areas, using the process established by FDA-led PFDD meetings as a model.[5] **Table 2** lists some examples of dermatologic conditions represented in FDA-led PFDD and patient organization–led PFDD meetings; note that this is not an exhaustive list.

In addition to FDA PFDD meetings, FDA is developing a series of 4 methodological PFDD guidance documents to facilitate systematic approaches to collect and use meaningful patient and caregiver input that can better inform medical product development and regulatory decision-making.

REGULATORY REVIEW OF CLINICAL OUTCOME ASSESSMENTS

For the regulatory review of COAs, such as PRO and ObsRO assessments, FDA focuses on whether the measure is fit for purpose[a]. Some general principles FDA uses to determine whether COAs are fit for purpose include the appropriateness of the assessment for its intended use (eg, study design, patient population); the ability of the assessment to validly and reliably measure concepts (eg, disease-related symptoms and impacts) that are clinically relevant, important to patients, and able to demonstrate change in a trial; and the ability for the COA data to be communicated in a way that is accurate, interpretable, and not misleading.

The FDA Guidance for Industry Patient-Reported Outcome Measures: Use in Medical Product Development to Support Labeling Claims can assist stakeholders in selecting and/or developing fit-for-purpose COAs.[8] Although the Guidance was developed for PRO assessments, many aspects of good measurement principles can be applied to development of other types of COAs such as ClinRO and ObsRO assessments.

CHALLENGES AND OPPORTUNITIES IN CAPTURING THE PATIENT VOICE IN DERMATOLOGIC CLINICAL TRIALS

Within dermatology drug development there are challenges in capturing the patient voice in certain dermatologic indications, such as those that involve pediatric populations and/or rare dermatologic conditions. Some of the challenges include but are not limited to the following:

- Fit-for-purpose rare disease- or pediatric-specific instruments do not exist for many conditions.

---

[a]The term fit for purpose is defined as a conclusion that the level of validation associated with a medical product development tool is sufficient to support its context of use (FDA-NIH Biomarker Working Group, 2016).

- Rare diseases can present with heterogenous signs, symptoms, and impacts.
- Instruments may not be sensitive to track children throughout their development.
- Vocabulary, numeracy, and comprehension of health concepts may be difficult in younger ages.
- The reliability and validity of self-report may be limited in young children.
- Inability to directly assess unobservable concepts (symptoms) in children who cannot self-report.

As stakeholders work to overcome these challenges, we encourage them to plan for early interactions with FDA to obtain feedback about their COA measurement strategy and collaboration within the precompetitive setting (eg, through consortia). Collaboration with FDA outside drug development, such as through the COA Qualification Program, may be another option[b]. The COA Qualification Program manages the qualification process for COAs intended to address unmet public health needs. COA qualification is a regulatory conclusion that the COA is a well-defined and reliable assessment of a specified concept of interest for use in adequate and well-controlled studies in a specified context of use.[9] Within the qualification program, FDA provides advice on the development or modification of COAs. Seeking qualification of a COA for a specified context of use, however, is voluntary. COAs that have not undergone the formal regulatory qualification procedure may still be used in regulatory applications, when scientifically appropriate for a specific application, based on agreement with the appropriate review division or office.[9]

An additional strategy to address these challenges may be to look to innovative approaches to COA. With the widespread adoption of smartphones, tablets, and other smart devices, mobile apps can provide a new platform to incorporate the patient perspective. Use of digital health technology in the form of sensors may allow us to assess important concepts such as sleep disruption and scratching behavior that indicate itch. Remote data capture can provide an opportunity to enhance implementation of endpoints that matter to patients in their lived experience, in part by allowing us to conduct more frequent assessments during periods between clinic visits. It also holds potential to reduce the barriers to clinical trial participation (eg, need for traveling for in person assessments), ultimately enabling more inclusive and generalizable trials.

Other opportunities to integrate the patient voice in dermatologic clinical trials may be through the exploration of other concepts beyond symptoms (eg, itch, skin pain), such as the impacts of the health condition. As exemplified by patient and caregiver input from PFDD meetings, many dermatologic conditions can have profound negative impact on patients' lives in areas such as physical and emotional functioning. For example, there are conditions that are not only symptomatic but also interfere with physical function and/or mobility (eg, conditions involving wounds or blisters, such as epidermolysis bullosa and pachyonychia congenita), as well as conditions that have emotional or psychological effects (eg, conditions that may cause social embarrassment and/or anxiety, such as hidradenitis suppurativa, hyperhidrosis, and others).

SUMMARY

Integrating the patient voice in clinical trials is critical in systematically capturing the patient experience, as well as determining successful treatment outcomes, particularly in dermatology. Patients' views of their signs and symptoms and how they may affect their daily lives are instrumental in treatment decisions in dermatology. FDA encourages the inclusion of PRO assessments and other types of COAs, where applicable, in clinical trials for emerging dermatology products. Incorporating measures that matter to patients allows the evaluation of the benefits and risks of new products from a patient-centered perspective and ultimately supports well-informed decision-making by patients and prescribers at the point of care.

DISCLAIMER STATEMENT

The views expressed in this publication are those of the authors and do not necessarily represent an official FDA position.

DISCLOSURE

All authors are employed by the U.S. government and report no conflicts of interest.

REFERENCES

1. Copley-Merriman C, Zelt S, Clark M, et al. Impact of measuring patient-reported outcomes in dermatology drug development. Patient 2017;10(2):203–13. Available at: https://doi-org.ezproxylocal.library.nova.edu/10.1007/s40271-016-0196-6.

---

[b]In Dec 2016, Congress passed the 21st Century Cures Act which then formalized the qualification process.

2. Mori S, Lee EH. Beyond the physician's perspective: a review of patient-reported outcomes in dermatologic surgery and cosmetic dermatology. Int J Womens Dermatol 2018;5(1):21–6. Available at: https://doi-org.ezproxylocal. library.nova.edu/10.1016/j.ijwd.2018.08.001.

3. FDA, Guidance for Industry, Food and Drug Administration Staff, and Other Stakeholders: Patient-Focused Drug Development: Collecting Comprehensive and Representative Input, June 2020a.

4. FDA, Guidance for Industry, Food and Drug Administration Staff, and Other Stakeholders: Patient-Focused Drug Development: Methods to Identify What Is Important to Patients, February 2022.

5. FDA. CDER Patient-Focused Drug Development. Available at: https://www.fda.gov/drugs/development-approval-process-drugs/cder-patient-focused-drug-development. Accessed April 5, 2021a.

6. FDA-NIH Biomarker Working Group. "BEST (biomarkers, EndpointS, and other tools) 516 resource," glossary. 2016. Available at: https://www.ncbi.nlm. nih.gov/books/NBK338448.

7. Townshend AP, Chen CM, Williams HC. How prominent are patient-reported outcomes in clinical trials of dermatological treatments? Br J Dermatol 2008;159(5): 1152–9. Available at: https://doi-org.ezproxylocal. library.nova.edu/10.1111/j.1365-2133.2008.08799.x.

8. FDA, Guidance for Industry, Patient-Reported Outcome Measures: Use in Medical Product Development to Support Labeling Claims, December 2009.

9. FDA, Guidance for Industry, Qualification Process for Drug Development Tools, November 2020b.

Moving?

Make sure your subscription moves with you!

To notify us of your new address, find your **Clinics Account Number** (located on your mailing label above your name), and contact customer service at:

Email: journalscustomerservice-usa@elsevier.com

800-654-2452 (subscribers in the U.S. & Canada)
314-447-8871 (subscribers outside of the U.S. & Canada)

Fax number: 314-447-8029

Elsevier Health Sciences Division
Subscription Customer Service
3251 Riverport Lane
Maryland Heights, MO 63043

*To ensure uninterrupted delivery of your subscription,
please notify us at least 4 weeks in advance of move.

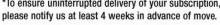

Printed and bound by CPI Group (UK) Ltd, Croydon, CR0 4YY

08/05/2025

01864704-0012